W9-AXZ-430

Building Your Nursing Career

A Guide for Students

Third Edition

JANICE WADDELL, RN, PhD
GAIL J. DONNER, RN, PhD
MARY M. WHEELER, RN, MEd, PCC

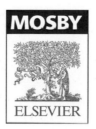

MOSBY

ELSEVIER

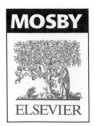

Copyright © 2009 Elsevier Canada, a division of Reed Elsevier Canada Ltd.

All rights reserved. No part of this publication may be reproduced or transmitted in any form or by any means, electronic or mechanical, including photocopy, recording, or any information storage and retrieval system, without permission in writing from the publisher. Reproducing passages from this book without such written permission is an infringement of copyright law.

Requests for permission to make any copies of any part of the work should be mailed to: College Licensing Officer, access ©, 1 Yonge Street, Suite 1900, Toronto, ON, M5E 1E5. Fax: (416) 868-1621. All other inquiries should be directed to the publisher.

Every reasonable effort has been made to acquire permission for copyright material used in this text and to acknowledge all such indebtedness accurately. Any errors and omissions called to the publisher's attention will be corrected in future printings.

Library and Archives Canada Cataloguing in Publication
Waddell, Janice, 1955–

    Building your nursing career: a guide for students / Janice
Waddell, Gail J. Donner, Mary M. Wheeler. – 3rd ed.
ISBN 978-1-897422-15-1

    1. Nursing – Vocational guidance. 2. Career development.
I. Donner, Gail J. (Gail Judith), 1942– II. Wheeler, Mary M. III. Title.
RT82.W32 2008   610.7306'9   C2008-901642-4

VP, Publishing: Ann Millar
Managing Developmental Editor: Martina van de Velde
Managing Production Editor: Rohini Herbert
Copy Editor: Michael Peebles
Cover Design: Gary Holgate
Interior Design: Monica Kompter
Typesetting and Assembly: Norm Reid
Printing and Binding: Transcontinental

Elsevier Canada
905 King Street West, 4th Floor, Toronto, ON, Canada M6K 3G9
Phone: 1-866-896-3331
Fax: 1-866-359-9534

Working together to grow
libraries in developing countries
www.elsevier.com | www.bookaid.org | www.sabre.org

ELSEVIER   BOOK AID International   Sabre Foundation

4 5   15 14 13

Contents

About the Authors

Janice Waddell, RN, PhD, is an associate professor at The Daphne Cockwell School of Nursing, Ryerson University, Toronto, Ontario. She is currently the Associate Dean for the Faculty of Community Services at Ryerson. Janice's clinical expertise is in the area of child and family violence. Her research foci include career planning and development for nurses (with a particular emphasis on student nurses and nursing faculty), the health experience of aggressive children, and children who have witnessed family violence. She teaches in both the undergraduate and graduate nursing programs at Ryerson University, focusing on advanced nursing education and professional issues and trends. Janice has facilitated numerous student-focused career planning and development workshops across Canada. She has been an associate of donnerwheeler since 1994.

Gail J. Donner, RN, PhD, is a partner in **donnerwheeler**, a consulting company focusing on career planning and development for health care professionals and health care organizations. Gail is a Professor and Dean Emeritus of the Lawrence S. Bloomberg Faculty of Nursing, University of Toronto, and active in nursing, in health care, and in her community.

Mary M. Wheeler, RN, MEd, PCC, is the other half of the **donnerwheeler** partnership. Mary is a certified coach with over 15 years of consulting expertise in career, organization, and human resource development and has published extensively with Gail in the area of career development, coaching, and mentoring.

Reviewers

Stephanie Buckingham, CD, RN, BSN, MA
Vancouver Island University
Nanaimo, British Columbia

Jim Hunter, RN, MSN
British Columbia Institute of Technology (BCIT)
Burnaby, British Columbia

Verna C. Pangman, RN, MEd, MN
University of Manitoba
Winnipeg, Manitoba

Tracie Risling, BA, BSN, MN, RN
Saskatchewan Institute of Applied Science and Technology (SIAST), Kelsey Campus
Saskatoon, Saskatchewan

D. Shane Strickland, RN, MScN
Lakehead University
Thunder Bay, Ontario

Career Planning and Development as a Student Activity

Welcome to *Building Your Nursing Career*. The rapidly changing world of health care offers tremendous opportunities as well as significant challenges to nursing students. They now learn in a variety of professional practice settings and thus have a first-hand look at nurses who work alone, with other nurses, or in interprofessional teams in roles as clinicians, educators, researchers, consultants, or managers. Changes in nursing and the health care system have created an environment in which individuals must become career resilient and self-directed and take control of their careers and futures. Developing the skills necessary for career resilience is a process that nursing students should engage in as soon as they begin their education.

Career resilience is about flexibility and adaptability. As a career-resilient student nurse, you seek and take advantage of meaningful and career-enhancing experiences both in the classroom and in nursing practice settings. You develop a growing sense of who you are as a nursing professional and are able to develop incrementally as you move through your educational program. Career-resilient students are dedicated to the idea of continuous learning and stand ready to re-invent themselves to keep pace with change. Moreover, career resilience conforms to the many definitions of nursing professional practice that include autonomy, self-direction, and continual learning.

In your student role, you are exposed to a wide range of practice settings and learn about many theoretical and technological advances as well as the current issues in nursing, the health care system, and society as a whole. In the midst of all your discoveries, it is often easy to lose sight of the career goals and aspirations that brought you to nursing. You may need and want help to plan and develop your career so that you orchestrate, rather than merely accumulate, your learning experiences.

How can I plan my career? What are the opportunities today, and what will they be in the future? How can I best use my educational experiences to advance my career goals? How can I be employable one year or several years from now? Who can help me? These are the questions student nurses are asking. You came to nursing with dreams, goals, and ideas about your future. You need a process to guide you in achieving your maximum potential as a student nurse so that you can actualize your dreams or alter them in response to your growing nursing experience and identification. Career planning and development is a dynamic process that adapts to the changes you will encounter as you build your nursing knowledge and experience.

The purposes of *Building Your Nursing Career* are two-fold: (1) to enhance your awareness of career planning and development and its importance today and in the future, and (2) to introduce you to a career planning and development model and a variety of career planning and development activities you can use throughout your nursing career. This guide is intended to provide you with the skills you need to build your career in nursing. We hope you find it informative and useful.

HOW TO USE YOUR STUDENT GUIDE

This guide introduces you to the Donner–Wheeler Career Planning and Development Model, referred to from now on as "the Model" (Figure 1–1). This Model is a tool you can use throughout your nursing education to develop as a professional and to build your career in a meaningful way. Each phase of the Model (scanning, assessing, visioning, planning, and marketing) is described along with specific activities and exercises to help you develop the skill to use the Model at all points in your educational program and later through the other stages of your career. You can use the Model to develop your nursing practice learning plans, select courses, determine foci for course assignments, engage in extracurricular activities and, most importantly, experience a sense of control over your academic career. Try to encourage your student colleagues to work together as you engage in the career planning and development process. As peers, you can offer each other support, feedback, and affirmation as you build your careers.

FIGURE 1-1
The Donner-Wheeler Career Planning and Development Model.

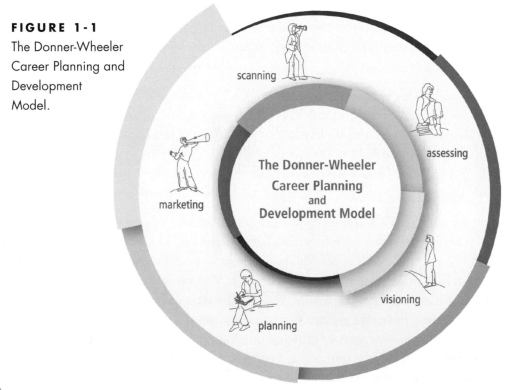

Your first step should be to read about each phase of the Model—what it is, why it is important, and how to use it. Then turn to the activities at the end of each phase and complete the questions. Each activity will help you tailor the career-building process to your own situation. As you become comfortable with the process, you will be able to move back and forth with ease among the five phases as you gather new experiences, skills, and knowledge.

This guide is primarily for undergraduate students who are entering nursing for the first time. However, the process and exercises provided are relevant to all nursing program and nursing education experiences. To learn more about the Model and the career planning and development process, read *Taking Control of Your Nursing Career*, 2nd edition, which is aimed at nurses at all stages of their careers; this book will serve as an informative and helpful resource for you as you progress through your nursing career.

As you begin the career planning and development process, you may wish to consider developing an electronic portfolio ("e-portfolio") to record your career planning and development activities. A portfolio can also help you reflect on your career achievements and successes as you work with the Model over the course of your academic program. The e-portfolio is technology based and can contain a significant amount of diverse information, including pictures, artwork, writing, sound, video, and creative graphics. If you are not familiar with e-portfolios, you can use the Internet to explore this concept and various ways to develop your professional Web portfolio (e-portfolio) by using a search engine such as "Google" and typing the terms "e-portfolio" or "web portfolio."

CAREER PLANNING AND DEVELOPMENT

A career is described as one's chosen profession, path, or course of life work. Students often think that their nursing career starts at the completion of their educational program and that active involvement in career planning becomes important only as they near graduation. In fact, you have chosen a path; your career has already started! You made an important life decision and began your professional career in nursing the day you registered for nursing courses. The career planning and development model presented in this guide provides you with a process by which you can develop your unique career goals and influence your educational activities to help you succeed in achieving your goals—regardless of where you are in your nursing program.

WHY CAREER PLANNING AND DEVELOPMENT IS IMPORTANT FOR NURSING STUDENTS

Nursing students are at various stages of entering a health care system that offers incredibly diverse opportunities for professional practice. Students describe feeling both excited and anxious when faced with the range of possibilities open to them—both in clinical placement settings and in their future nursing practice. As John, a fourth-year nursing student, observed:

"I am currently completing a very important phase of my life by graduating. At the same time, I will be entering one of the most exciting phases by officially starting a career in nursing. What I am realizing is that I am the only one responsible for my career. Opportunities will not simply fall into my hands; rather, I need to take charge and control my professional future through career planning. I know there are lots of jobs out there; I want to make sure I accept a job that is right for me and fits with my career plans."

Although at a different level in her nursing education program, Leah, a second-year student, described similar feelings:

"I've just finished my second year, and I feel like I now have only 2 years left to make sure I get all of the experience I can to be marketable when I graduate. I'm not sure what my goals are or how I can "work the system" to make sure I get what I need."

The career planning process can serve as a guide to help students to achieve a sense of control and focus related to their educational activities and to prepare for future employment. The career planning and development process helps students to answer the following questions:

✦ Where have I been (before nursing school and over the course of my program)?
✦ Where am I now? What am I learning, and what are my interests?
✦ Where would I like to go? What are my hopes for my next step in my education and for my future practice?
✦ How will I get there? How can I plan my courses and make the best of my clinical placements so that I can move toward my goals?

The answers to these questions will be quite different for students at varying stages in their education.

JOHN Over the course of his nursing education, John (the fourth-year student) accumulated a solid foundation of nursing practice experiences and professional courses. As a result, his responses to these questions will reflect a wide range of nursing-related knowledge and experience.

LEAH Leah (the second-year student) may not have the same breadth of nursing practice experience and range of course work as John, but she can build on her beginning foundation in nursing, her life experiences, and her hopes and dreams for her professional education. Reflecting on these questions can help Leah acknowledge all that she has brought to the profession and how her nursing education can serve to guide her future plans.

Regardless of where you are in your educational program, the career planning process involves thought, insight, and dedicated time. Although many resources are available for you to use in planning your career, the one most important to your career development is you! The career planning and development process is really about developing a life skill—one that you can apply not only in your educational and professional endeavours but also in your personal life.

THE DONNER-WHEELER CAREER PLANNING AND DEVELOPMENT MODEL

Career development is not a one-time activity, nor do you need to follow a step-by-step process. Once you have worked through the Model, you can move back and forth among the phases, adding and changing the content of your insights, information, and plans to reflect your developing nursing practice. The Model allows you to track your progress in your professional growth in nursing and to plan for your upcoming learning activities. In your educational program, you have built-in cues about when to "check in" with your career development. End of terms, evaluation times, and the development of learning plans are transition times that you can use to guide and build on your work with the career model. The career development process will prompt you to do the following:

1. Understand and use the environment around you to develop your nursing career.
2. Assess your growing strengths and development needs and validate that assessment.
3. Envision what your nursing career can be.
4. Develop a plan for using your educational activities in a way that will help you move toward your career vision.
5. Market yourself to achieve your career vision and related career goals.

Career development helps you stay focused and challenged so that you can create learning opportunities related to your goals or find meaning in experiences that, at face value, do not seem relevant or responsive to your immediate learning needs. The five phases of the Model include the items listed in the box below.

The Donner-Wheeler Career Planning and Development Model

Scanning Your Environment
What are the current realities and future trends?

Completing Your Self-Assessment and Reality Check
Who am I?
How do others see me?

Creating Your Career Vision
What do I really want to be doing?

Developing Your Strategic Career Plan
How can I achieve my career goals?

Marketing Yourself
How can I best market myself?

2

Planning Your Career

Y ou are now ready to learn to use the Donner-Wheeler Career Planning and Development Model (the Model). This chapter provides you with the details of each of the Model's five phases, along with examples from student lives and experiences. We have included activities to help you apply the Model to your particular educational level and personal and professional goals. Take time to review each phase carefully, and then proceed with the exercises. Remember, this is not a one-time activity but something you will want and need to come back to as you progress through your program and as your environment, experience, and interests change.

You can begin your work at any phase of the Model. Some nurses find it helpful to begin with scanning their environment to explore what is "out there" with a focus on expanding their practice or choosing a new direction in their nursing career. Others choose to begin with their self-assessment as a strategy to reflect on, and articulate, their current strengths, areas for development, and recent accomplishments and follow this reflection with a scan of their environment with an eye to finding a fit between the outcome of their self-assessment and existing opportunities.

We have found that students find their initial work with the Model most exciting if they begin with creating their career vision. You begin with giving yourself the freedom to dream about what and who you wish to look like in the future.

CREATING YOUR CAREER VISION

What Is a Career Vision?

Your career vision describes where you want to go in your nursing career and how you wish to fulfill your nursing role; it is a description of you and what you wish to become. Your vision allows you to imagine what is possible and serves as a guide to how you can orchestrate your educational experiences to help you meet your career goals. Your vision can focus on who and what you wish to be in your nursing career. Regardless of the focus, your vision provides you with a purpose and some insights into what you need to achieve your dream.

Why Should I Have a Career Vision?

Having a career vision is perhaps the most forceful motivator for using your nursing practice placement and classroom experiences and your summer and part-time work opportunities to the fullest. Your vision can help you focus on how you can make the best of your learning opportunities rather than just reacting to events as they occur. Creating a career vision answers the question, "What do I want?" With an idea of what you would like your career to look like, you can approach any course or nursing practice placement with a sense of how it may help you get where you want to go. With each new encounter you have with the world of nursing, your career vision may alter or perhaps change altogether. Therefore, you should continually ask yourself, "Am I still feeling the way I felt about nursing when I entered my nursing program? Does my career vision still reflect who and what I wish to be?" You can use a journal to continue to explore and reflect on this question as you move along in your nursing program and your nursing career. As a matter of fact, this would be a good time to begin keeping a journal of your thoughts and dreams. A journal is a powerful tool for keeping track of where you are headed and all the ideas and plans you have for getting there. It is your private record of who you are, what is important to you, and how you are changing. Many people have found a journal to be a valuable resource for "sorting things out."

Student nurses are often uncertain about how they can design their career futures while still in their educational program. Just as with courses, it is unlikely that individual students have their choice of where they will have their nursing practice experiences, nor can they select all of their courses to suit their current interests. However, students can approach any nursing practice setting, classroom environment, or work or volunteer experience with focused goals that will help them progress toward their career vision. These personal learning goals may be an added dimension to the learning that is structured through the curriculum. Often, it is in nursing practice settings that are seemingly unrelated to their career visions that students can be the most creative and active in shaping their learning. Many students find that when they optimize opportunities, as opposed to resisting the unknown, they end up discovering more choices than they had ever considered.

We suggest that you save your career vision in an electronic file. Print it, and place it where you can see it on a regular basis—most likely near your computer screen! Each time you sit down to contemplate an assignment, develop your learning plan, or update your self-assessment, use your vision to guide your work and your focus. How can you best use your curricular activities to help you progress toward your vision? Be active in shaping your academic activities to ensure that they are helping you achieve your career vision. Keeping your vision close at hand also helps you recognize whether your vision is still what you wish it to be or if your recent experiences require that you either change it or further affirm that it remains true to your dream. At any time in your academic career, you may have more than one career vision or your vision may change as you gather diverse experiences and opportunities. Career visions are not written in stone; if elements of your vision change over time or you have a complete shift to a new vision, you can use the Model to help you utilize what you have accomplished to create new opportunities and directions.

Caroline created her career vision by using the questions outlined above as she began the third year of her nursing program. Through the process of creating her vision, Caroline realized that she had a dream for her career that she had not articulated, even to herself.

> I guess in the back of my mind I have always thought I would like to go to Africa and work in a community-based clinic. Walking through the questions to develop my vision, I realized that this is what I want to aim for and that I can start now to set myself up to actually do it. I feel an excitement and a sense of optimism about my future career that I have not felt for a while.

Caroline had developed an e-portfolio to help her keep track of her vision and other phases of the Model and included a picture of an African village to remind herself why she is doing what she is doing and where she hopes to go. She printed both her written vision and the picture so that they were in view when she worked at her computer.

JALYNN Jalynn, a second-year student, has a career vision that centres on her dream of being a maternal–child nurse. Her practice placement was in a mental health setting, and she expressed concern that she would need to put her hopes for a maternal–child nursing focus "on hold" during this placement experience. In spite of a seeming lack of fit between her career vision as an expert maternal–child nurse and the area of mental health, she shared her vision with both her nursing practice instructor and her preceptor. She also met with her faculty mentor, who has expertise in maternal–child nursing. She was reminded by each of these resources that she could focus her learning goals on communication skills and family-centred care and could request to work with any pregnant women admitted to her placement setting. At the end of term, Jalynn evaluated her mental health experience as a most valuable learning experience in terms of refining her therapeutic communication skills with both short-term and long-term clients and their families. She also discovered that the competencies she strengthened during this experience would serve her well when working with new mothers and families, something she also found that she could articulate.

How to Create Your Own Career Vision

Creating a career vision involves *affirmation* (composing a statement of what you want to create in your life), *visualization* (forming a picture or image of what you want to create), and *germination* (being committed to a vision you believe will be realized). It begins with taking time to do some active daydreaming about an ideal day in your future. Your career vision will be as individual as you are. To create it, you will need to ask yourself some important questions and give yourself permission to let go of what you previously thought possible.

Two general questions will guide you in this process. The questions "What do I want?" and "What am I seeking?" help you get started—rather like a warm-up or brainstorming session. No answer is wrong. The questions "What is my ideal vision for my career?" and "What would my ideal day look like?" provide more focus as you begin to create your career vision. Formulate your career vision in the present tense, as if it were occurring right now, and formulate it in as much descriptive detail as possible.

SANDEEP Sandeep, a second-year nursing student, had just completed his final nursing practice placement of the year in a medical-surgical unit. He found that in his last placement, he enjoyed working with younger patients, especially an adolescent with a recent diagnosis of cancer. He was able to work with the adolescent and her family for a few weeks and received feedback that he made a positive difference in the hospital experience of this family.

Sandeep, described his career vision as follows:

"I am an expert advanced practice nurse at an active pediatric oncology unit in a large teaching hospital located in a metropolitan city. I feel confident working with children and families who are experiencing cancer, and I feel that I serve as a resource and clinical expert for my nursing colleagues. I am seen by my colleagues as knowledgeable, approachable, and supportive. The hospital in which I work supports my ongoing learning and my practice. Families feel they can trust me to advocate for their needs and to involve them in all aspects of their care. I leave each day feeling I have made a difference to children and families experiencing cancer. When I arrive home, I have the energy to connect with my friends and family."

Although Sandeep was aware that his ultimate career vision might change as he encountered new areas of professional practice, he developed a vision that reflected his current hopes and dreams.

A third-year student created a career vision statement that reflected her progressive interest in community health nursing:

In one of my first-year nursing courses, a nurse who worked solely with the homeless population in our city spoke to the class about her nursing experiences. I was hooked! I decided right then that I wanted my nursing practice to centre on caring for homeless clients. I created my career vision and have used my nursing practice and course experiences to help me prepare to achieve my goals. I also asked a nurse who works exclusively with the homeless population in my area to be my mentor. Although my vision changes slightly as I learn more about myself, nursing, and the health care system, the essence of my vision has remained fairly constant.

Career Vision: I am an expert community-based nurse with recognized expertise in the needs and care of individuals and groups who live on the streets of large urban centres. I lobby on both local and national levels and serve as a resource to my nursing colleagues, health care policymakers, and the media. I work with an interdisciplinary team that values the contributions of each team member. My employers support my work with the homeless population and my efforts to be an effective advocate and lobbyist. I know that I make a difference to individuals, and, together with my supportive colleagues, I can make a difference at a broader level. At the end of the day, I return home to my family with a sense of accomplishment and anticipation.

Your career vision does not need to be specific to a specialty area of nursing (e.g., pediatrics, emergency, intensive care, community health). Your vision can articulate the type of professional you wish to be. For example, a first-year student developed the following career vision:

Career Vision: I am an expert nurse who is recognized for my extensive knowledge base, my exceptional interpersonal skills, my clinical practice excellence, and my commitment to collaborative practice. My colleagues describe me as the person you want to have around when you are working—supportive, knowledgeable, kind, and accessible. I have fun at work and trust that my colleagues share my commitment to working toward the highest quality of care possible. I end my day knowing that I have done excellent work and ready to enjoy an evening with my partner.

Lydia, a fourth-year student, looked to her nursing practice placement experiences as a means to explore a number of career options. Her career vision reflected her desire to be an entrepreneur in her still undecided nursing practice specialty:

Career Vision: I am an independent nursing practitioner with specific research and practice expertise working in a consulting role. I work with individual clients and organizations to establish and evaluate programs in my area of nursing practice expertise. I am recognized for my knowledge, skill, and ability to work effectively and efficiently to produce a relevant "product" of excellent quality. I am known for my collaborative approach to projects and my commitment to ensuring that the work that we do makes a difference to the stakeholders. At the end of each day, I am confident that I have given my all to a project and have learned something new. I head to the gym and then home, where my dog and two cats are waiting for me!

Whether your career vision involves a clinical nursing practice specialty, a professional image, or both, it can serve as a motivating guide as you progress toward your dream.

Now you are ready to develop your career vision. Do Activity 1.

Activity (1) Creating Your Career Vision

When you start, your vision does not need to be perfectly realistic; that comes later in the process, when you set your career goals. Do not worry about your vision being too big, too vague, or too impossible. It should be grand and inspiring; if it is an important dream, it may even be a little scary.

Now, close your eyes, put your feet up, and picture yourself as a nurse doing exactly what you want to do where you want to do it and doing it well! Imagine yourself on a typical day, heading off to your ideal nursing position in the workplace that allows you to do the best job possible. Use the following questions to guide your visioning exercise.

➢ Where do you live?

➢ What is the weather like as you head into work?

➢ How are you getting to work (e.g., walking, driving, cycling, or public transit)?

➤ How do you feel as you head into your work day?

➤ What does the building in which you work look like? How does your workplace support you and your nursing practice?

➤ When you get to work, you overhear a colleague who knows you well describing you to a nurse just starting her employment. What words does your colleague use to describe you?

➤ As you enter the area where your clients are, what kind of work will you be doing, and how do your clients perceive you?

➢ Who works most closely with you? How does your organization support your work?

➢ As you head home at the end of your day, how do you feel about what you have accomplished?

➢ What or who awaits you at the end of your day?

What Have You Accomplished?

You have a dream! This dream may change over the course of your educational program, or it may stay with you until your graduation. Either way, your dream can help you create and use your future learning activities. Your dream is your guide.

SCANNING YOUR ENVIRONMENT

What Is Scanning?

Scanning the environment involves simply looking around with the goal of identifying how your immediate and surrounding environment can help you work toward your career vision. You have already been introduced to the process of scanning the environment as a nursing student. As you learn to plan and deliver nursing care, you also learn to observe your client's environment and the variables that influence the client's health status (e.g., resources, social factors, economic realities). Your nursing curriculum also offers you structured opportunities, usually in classes and seminars, to learn about important elements of an environmental scan, such as current issues in nursing, health care, work design, and society at large. Each of these elements are important to consider within the context of your career vision.

Scanning the environment and then identifying your own strengths and interests will give you the information you need to help you identify possibilities for your current and future nursing practice experiences, professional skill development, and course selection. It helps you answer the following questions:

✦ What opportunities are available that would help me progress toward my career vision?
✦ What do I need to be aware of?
✦ What and who are my resources?

The breadth of your environmental scan may vary depending on where you are in your nursing program. In the early years of your program, you may find it most helpful to concentrate your scan on your school, curriculum requirements, nursing practice placement settings, and the information available through these resources. In the first and second years of your program, the primary focus of your scan is likely to be on discovering and on using the school environment to your best advantage. As you advance, you will be looking toward preparing for graduation and entry to practice. Your preparation will rely on greater knowledge of what is happening outside your immediate learning environment. Extending your scan to include learning about health care and nursing-specific issues and trends locally, provincially, nationally, and even internationally will be an important next step.

Students are at a definite advantage when doing environmental scans. You have ready access to this information from your course work, faculty members, and nursing practice agencies. Using the scan to help you with your career planning is just another way to apply your learning. You are already ahead of the game!

Why Is Scanning Important?

Scanning helps you discover opportunities and resources within your nursing program as well as current and future employment opportunities. Your career vision reminds you of who and where you hope to be in the future. The process of scanning can help you make the best of your learning experiences and identify both short- and long-term goals and learning activities in keeping with your career vision. Without continuous scanning, it is difficult to focus your development to your best advantage, difficult to know the best direction in which to head, and even more difficult to influence your learning activities and professional development.

How and When Do You Scan?

The simple answer is—continuously! You can scan throughout your educational program to learn what is happening now and what may happen in the future. Sources of information include the following:

✦ Course readings
✦ Discussions with faculty, preceptors, and mentors
✦ Professional and popular journals; printed and other forms of news media
✦ The Internet
✦ Observations
✦ Friends and colleagues
✦ Everyday experiences
✦ Professional organizations
✦ Unions

One student shares her feeling that her professional organization is a great source of information:

> I find it very helpful to read clips from my professional organization. After joining as a student member, I was sent regular newsletters and media clips via e-mail. I find that these clips are really helpful in keeping me up to speed on what is happening locally, nationally, and globally in the world of nursing—and how I can make a difference, even as a student.

Reading, talking, and listening are the means you will use to make sense of the information you collect. As a student, you have the added benefit of a number of faculty members, preceptors, mentors, and student colleagues who are "at your fingertips" to help you direct, interpret, and use the information you will collect in your scan. Once you have gathered all the information, it is helpful to organize it into school, local, national, and global categories. You can add information to these categories at any time.

You should think of your scan as a work in progress, something you continually update and revise to reflect your growing experience, knowledge, and understanding of the nursing world. Students often complete a scan with the broad goal of determining how they can best shape their nursing practice experiences and course selection to advance toward their career vision. Hence, they may concentrate their scan on local and school-related trends, issues, and resources. Students in the latter years of the program find that extending their focus to provincial (or state) and national levels gives them information they need to make decisions regarding what steps to take after graduation. The data from your scan can be guided by, and inform, your career vision. Whatever your vision and focus, try to make scanning an integral part of your everyday academic and personal life.

LAURA Laura, a third-year nursing student, first used the environmental scan to help her look at an upcoming nursing practice placement with a focus on how this experience could help her develop professional competencies required for her to achieve her vision of being a community health nurse in the area of child and family health. In the winter term, she was going to a gerontology-focused community health setting. She was interested in using her scan to help develop a clear focus for her learning plan for the coming term, one that would allow her to concentrate on overall learning goals in addition to the serendipitous learning that naturally occurs in a new placement setting.

Laura began her scan by obtaining a list of the course readings related to the community health course. A brief look at the readings gave her an idea of current issues and trends in community health nursing, both nationally and locally. She then met a faculty member with expertise in child and family community health nursing. Their discussion about the nature of community health nursing and nursing roles in community health helped her get a sense of what she could anticipate in her winter placement. Moreover, the faculty member was able to help Laura develop some learning goals that could be achieved within a gerontological community health setting that would also help her build professional competencies relevant to child and family health.

Finally, Laura phoned her contact person at the community placement setting and asked what she could do to prepare for her placement. With all of this information in hand, she decided on two broad learning goals: (1) developing knowledge and skill in community-based program planning and evaluation; and (2) strengthening her competencies in working within a family-centred care model in the community context. Her self-assessment would then help her identify her unique areas for development and specify learning objectives related to these goals.

Recall Caroline, the third-year student whose dream was to work in a community-based clinic in Africa. Caroline used her

Continued

vision to guide her environmental scan. She began her scan by checking her student handbook to find the research and clinical practice interests of her nursing faculty members. She discovered that a faculty member in her school of nursing was involved in research related to sustainable health programs in Africa. Caroline arranged a meeting with the faculty member; in their conversation, she shared her vision of working in an African community. Her faculty contact was able to direct Caroline to a colleague working at a teaching hospital nearby who was leading an African mission with a focus on nursing children with human immuno-deficiency virus. From that contact, Caroline was put in touch with two fourth-year students who had spent the previous summer doing volunteer health work in Africa.

Caroline's scan was not complicated; she focused on resources within her school of nursing and ended up with a rich array of contacts and information on how she could best use her courses and nursing practice placements to position her to develop competencies, in the short and long terms, that fit with her long-term vision. Her next step was to work on her self-assessment to determine how she could shape her learning experiences in the coming terms.

Now that you understand what scanning is and how to use it, try Activity 2.

Activity (2) Scanning Your Environment

The trends and issues you identify in your scan can help you make decisions about potential opportunities within your classroom and nursing practice environments. Use your career vision to develop additional questions to guide your scan. What do you need to know to develop specific career goals and learning objectives that will help you capitalize on opportunities within your academic activities? General questions may include the following.

➤ Is there someone who is the kind of nurse I hope to be or currently doing the type of work I would like to do ? What are the characteristics of that person or work?

➤ Are there environmental constraints I must consider when planning to do what I really want to do?

➤ What environmental supports or resources would facilitate my progress toward my career vision?

The following is a more detailed guide that can help you with your scan. Consider school, local, and national areas. If you feel ready to extend your scan to the global level, then include that category as well.

For each of the categories (school, local, national, global), consider issues related to society, to health in general, and to nursing, within the context of your vision. Insert those trends and issues you observe to be important at this time as you consider where you are in your development and where you hope to be in the future. To help you as you fill in your scan, we have provided you with some questions to consider and a sampling of possible answers. Your list of questions and answers will likely grow over time.

Remember that you will need to review and revise your scan on a regular basis. The end of each term can be a cue to update your scan.

SCHOOL

➢ What are some of the opportunities or realities of your school setting?
Examples: Components of the nursing curriculum, required courses, course electives, placement opportunities, faculty resources and mentors, student association representatives, interdisciplinary courses

LOCAL

➢ What are some of the important social and health issues in your local area?
Examples: Changing demographics of the client population, shift in care to the community, increasing caregiver burden, client and workplace safety, environment

➢ What are the important nursing issues in your local area?
Examples: Shortage or surplus of nurses, demographics (e.g., aging) of nurses, changing practice settings, changing roles in the practice setting

NATIONAL

➢ What are the significant national health and social trends?
Examples: Controlling health care costs, decreasing lengths of hospital stays, community-based care, infant mortality, increased use of technology

➢ What are the national issues affecting nurses?
Examples: Shortage of nurses, education specialization, quality of worklife

GLOBAL

➢ What health or social issues seem to be worldwide phenomena?
Examples: Infectious diseases, ethical issues, allocation of resources, the gap between rich and poor people, social determinants of health

➢ What nursing issues seem to be global in scope?
Examples: Recruitment and retention, regulation, quality of worklife, changing practice

Scanning Your Environment

School		
Curriculum/Courses	Placement Opportunities	Faculty Resources

Local Trends and Issues		
Society	Health Care	Nursing

National Trends and Issues		
Society	Health Care	Nursing

Global Trends and Issues		
Society	Health Care	Nursing

What Have You Accomplished?

You have a vision for your career. Completing an initial environmental scan has given you some valuable information about what is available in your school, the issues nurses currently face, the type of opportunities available for your course and nursing practice experiences, and how these opportunities can help you to achieve your vision. This information helps you to see what is possible and realistic so that you can make the best of your learning experiences.

What Is Your Next Step?

You now have a better understanding of the nursing and health care world. The next step is getting a sense of how your interests, values, and abilities fit with your hopes for the future. This process is called self-assessment. After completing the self-assessment, you should do a reality check of it with others.

COMPLETING YOUR SELF-ASSESSMENT AND REALITY CHECK

What Is Self-Assessment?

Your self-assessment helps you identify your values, experiences, knowledge, strengths, and areas for development and then link them with your career vision and environmental scan to plan the next educational steps you wish to take. Your self-assessment helps you shift your vision from the future to the present. When you scanned the environment, you focused on what surrounds you and on building an understanding of how that influences your present and future development. The self-assessment focuses on you. It can assist you in recognizing all the attributes that make you who you are, what areas you would like to focus on for further development, and what you have to offer. Your self-assessment also provides you with the opportunity to think about how your personal life goals influence, and are influenced by, your career vision and choices.

Completing your self-assessment and reality check will allow you to give honest and accurate answers to two questions: (1) Who am I? (2) How do others see me? When you put your self-assessment together with your vision and the results of your environmental scan, your answers will enable you to complete the last phases of the career planning and development process: developing your strategic career plan and marketing yourself to implement your plan.

Why Is Assessing Yourself Important?

As a student nurse, an awareness of your values, skills, and strengths will provide insight into what you have brought to the profession and what areas you would like to develop further. It forms an important basis for making plans and developing the type of career or future that is congruent with your vision and is what you want.

Some students believe they have no say in planning their educational experiences. It is true that nursing curricula, like those of other professional disciplines, have required courses and learning activities, and you may not have a choice about whether or not to take those courses. However, you can choose how to interpret and use these courses to meet your unique needs. In addition to the required courses, there is usually a range of elective courses from which you can select according to your interests and preferences. Within both scenarios, your ability to use your learning to meet your professional and personal learning needs (which, preferably, are similar) depends on how well you know yourself. Self-knowledge about interests, values, knowledge, skills, strengths, and limitations can help you look at any experience as a meaningful learning opportunity. Sharing your assessment helps others respond to your unique needs.

In many ways, as a nursing student, you have an advantage in this fundamental step of the career planning and development process. Most nursing curricula require that you participate in some form of self-reflection and self-evaluation. The key to success is to find meaning in the doing. Too often, nursing students approach the self-reflective process as an academic exercise rather than as a means of enhancing their own career development. Once you claim the process of reflection as your own, you will be able to capitalize on your identified strengths and life experiences across all dimensions of your educational experiences. Revisiting your career vision and self-assessment at the end of each term will allow you to update your knowledge of self, set new learning goals, and develop career goals and action plans that will contribute to your ability to advance toward your vision. Using your self-assessment to guide your participation in your curriculum will give you the confidence to find or create meaning in your future learning experiences.

During or prior to your nursing program, you may have used assessment tools such as the Myers-Briggs Type Inventory (a personality test), the Leadership 360 Assessment (an assessment that includes feedback from a number of sources, including fellow employees, supervisors, and others), and more general learning style inventories. If you have used these or other assessment tools, you may find such previous work helpful as you move forward on this phase of the Model.

Beginning the Self-Assessment Process

The first questions are "Who am I?" and "How would you describe yourself?" Answering these questions involves much more than describing what you do or where you are in your educational preparation. Even though you spend a considerable amount of time at school (and perhaps at work) to support your academic endeavours, it is important to acknowledge those other components that complete your life, including your personal health, well-being, and development; your family and friends; your community; and your personal life goals.

Although you may be new to nursing, you have had valuable life experiences prior to entering your nursing program that have contributed to your current strengths in nursing. For example, think about all the adjectives you could use to describe what makes you unique. Although we are all unique, the challenge lies in being able to articulate that uniqueness. Can you make a list of three characteristics that define your uniqueness? Think back to your visioning experience. Often the adjectives you envisioned your colleagues using to describe you reflect your current unique attributes. Pick up a pencil and paper and make that list—now! Keep that list, and refer to it and revise it from time to time. Who we are includes our beliefs and values, our knowledge and skills, our interests, and our hopes for our future. *Beliefs* are the way in which we view ourselves and the world around us. *Values* are a set of beliefs that drive our decisions, actions, reactions, behaviours, and relations. *Knowledge and skills* are the abilities and behaviours we use to produce results, and *interests* are the activities on which we like to spend most of our time and from which we gain pleasure.

Assessing Your Values

Values are those principles we prize and cherish—those beliefs we hold as extremely important. Values direct our decisions and influence our lives. As you begin to identify your values, consider why you chose nursing as a career and how your experiences to date fit with those values. Ask yourself the following questions:

✦ What is important to me in my educational and personal lives?
✦ What significant experiences or interests prompted me to consider nursing as a career?
✦ Who has inspired me in my nursing education, and what values did that person convey to me?
✦ What can I contribute to nursing?
✦ What values influence my learning and my development as a nurse?
✦ Who or what are the significant things in my life that I need to consider at this time?
✦ What are my priorities—self, partner, family, school, work, community, or other?

Read your career vision and identify the values that are embedded in that vision. Those values may relate to what you need to have in your workplace to be satisfied (e.g., support for ongoing learning, resources that allow you to offer a high quality of care, colleagues who share your commitment to quality care). Your vision may also highlight values related to your ability to make a difference, remain passionate about what you do, have fun, and experience a sense of collegiality. Your hopes for the future can offer you insight into what you value as an individual in the nursing profession.

If you find that you are having difficulty articulating your values, there are many resources that can help you with values clarification. The "Career Planning and Development Resources" section includes two online sources related to values clarification that may help you as you work on this important phase of your career planning and development.

MARIA   Maria recognized the strong influence her mother had on her choice of nursing as a career. Her mother, who had been a nurse, exemplified warmth, caring, and strength—the qualities Maria associated with nursing. In addition to demonstrating respect for the uniqueness and integrity of each individual, Maria's mother modelled the power of nursing to influence the quality of health care. She accomplished this through individual interactions both with clients and with her nursing colleagues. Her mother's willingness to campaign for those not able to advocate for themselves fostered the value Maria places on the importance of individual efforts in influencing the perceptions and actions of decision makers at all levels of health care.

Maria also had the opportunity to accompany her mother when she volunteered at a senior citizens home. During these visits, Maria directly observed the positive effect her mother and the other nurses had on the residents through their professional presence and individualized approach to care. Long-term exposure to this setting fostered Maria's interest in nursing as a career, with a vision of working with older adults in a complex long-term care environment. In addition, her teachers, family members, and friends told her that she was very good with people and would make a great nurse. Her vision of being a warm, caring, and committed professional interested in working closely with older adults helped Maria articulate her values and keep these in mind as she evaluated various practice experiences and other academic activities.

Maria states, "It's funny. I always knew I wanted to be a nurse, to make a difference in people's lives, but it wasn't until I sat down and really thought about why I wanted to be a nurse that I realized what an excellent role model my mom has been and how that modelling has influenced my decision to go into nursing, with a vision toward geriatric nursing. I can see how I have come to value many of the things my mom does and how these values will help me to be an effective nurse. I was also able to get a first-hand view of how rewarding it can be to care for this client population."

Assessing Your Knowledge and Skills

Career visions provide information regarding the breadth and depth of professional competencies you will require to actualize hopes for the future. The self-assessment process allows you to consider where you are at now, relative to where you are going.

Recognizing what knowledge and skills you possess—and to what degree you possess them—are crucial outcomes of the self-assessment process. Knowledge develops through a combination of formal learning and experience whereas skills are acquired abilities. By reviewing your past accomplishments, nursing practice and classroom evaluations, and nursing program goals, you can begin to identify your strengths and the areas you would like to develop further. Consider your career vision and the work you have done within your nursing program and in your non-nursing life. Your community and social environments also provide opportunities for acknowledging your current strengths and increasing your knowledge and skills about people and the world in which you live.

As you accumulate classroom and nursing practice experiences, you will gather current feedback related to your strengths, your progress, and areas to develop from a variety of instructors, peers, and nursing practice contacts. Share your vision with those who you think can help you assess your current strengths and who can assist you in targeting areas for development. Remember to seek and value feedback that relates to all of your professional competencies, not just your psychomotor skill set. In the past, job requirements tended to relate only to job duties or "hard skills" (e.g., those involved with providing direct nursing care to clients), not to work attitudes, general communication, and interpersonal skills. When you sit down to evaluate your professional competencies, take into account your personality and nature, your attitude, the way you work with others, and the ease with which you communicate. These attributes or "soft skills" are as important as your technical clinical nursing practice skills and often are highly transferable and highly valued by health care organizations.

Recognizing your knowledge and skill gaps or limitations is just as important as acknowledging your strengths. If you do not recognize these limitations, you may miss important learning opportunities.

You should ask yourself the following questions:

✦ What knowledge and skills did I bring with me when I entered my nursing program?
✦ What knowledge and skills have I developed, both personally and professionally?
✦ What are my strengths?
✦ What are my limitations?
✦ What knowledge and skills require further development?

Many of the successes and strengths you have enjoyed in other areas of your life will hold you in good stead in your nursing career. If you are in the first year of your nursing program, start by considering your past accomplishments with a focus on the values, insight, skills, and strengths that you developed as a result of your efforts.

DOMINIC Dominic's career vision focused on working with a neonatal intensive care transport team. He wished to be considered a valued, resourceful, and committed member of the transport team.

Dominic identified his involvement on the high school rowing team as an accomplishment. When he focused on the skills he had developed as a result of this experience, he identified strengths in team-work, an ability to successfully balance academic and extracurricular activities, and skill in coaching new team members effectively. Reflecting on his positive experiences with his rowing team also helped Dominic realize how much he valued working as part of a team. Each of these skills and insights would be an asset to him while participating in his academic career with an eye on his vision.

INDIRA Indira's career vision placed her in the role of an expert pediatric nurse working in an acute care teaching hospital. She saw herself involved in the direct care of children and families and as a resource to her colleagues.

Indira was employed as a nanny for three young children during the summer months. She was able to identify her knowl-edge of the developmental issues and needs of the preschool and school-aged child, the enjoyment she experienced when working with children, and her strengths in the areas of organization, patience, and perseverance. Indira also noted how her experience as a nanny heightened her awareness of the importance of family in the lives of children.

After identifying their strengths and skills, students can focus on enhancing them in the context of their nursing experience by asking for specific feedback and seeking experiences to meet their unique learning needs. Awareness of their values can also add insight and clarity to their reflection and evaluation of each learning experience. Students can use the journalizing process to reflect on the impact of their experiences on their evolving professional practice competencies, and their career vision can foster a sense of focus and progress.

Assessing Your Interests

Interests provide another guide in determining your current and future learning goals and in deciding how you would ideally like to meet those goals. They can be grouped into four categories:

✦ People: helping, serving, caring for, or selling things to people
✦ Data: working with facts, records, or files
✦ Things: working with machines, tools, or living things such as plants and animals
✦ Ideas: creating insights, theories, or new ways of saying or doing something

What have you liked about your past jobs and current job, summer employment, part-time jobs, academic jobs (e.g., research assistant, work-study student), or volunteer activities? What did you dislike? In what type of environment do you learn and perform at your best? What do you like to do outside of the academic environment or your current workplace? What energizes or motivates you? Answering these questions will help you understand and articulate your interests.

Recognizing Your Accomplishments

Accomplishments are those specific successes that have marked the highlights of your performance in any of your roles (e.g., as student nurse, volunteer, or employee). For example, you may have developed a client teaching package, provided an in-service for the staff at your nursing practice placement, or received acknowledgement or recognition for your strong communication or leadership skills in your student role. These accomplishments represent those times in your life when you made a difference. They become the added value you will bring to any nursing practice environment.

JACOB Jacob, a fourth-year student, was in the process of planning his final-year nursing practice placements. His career vision focused on the kind of nurse he wished to be as opposed to a specific practice specialty. He admired nurses who could really focus on the people with whom they worked—clients, families, and colleagues. He also strove to emulate nurses who could establish positive and meaningful relationships while simultaneously providing exceptional physical care. His vision was to be that kind of nurse; he was just unsure of where to do so.

A detailed self-assessment was invaluable to Jacob. He was undecided about whether he should request a medical-surgical setting or a long-term care setting. While completing his self-assessment, he discovered that he (1) valued the continuity of working with adult clients experiencing chronic illness, (2) was interested in working with people over time, (3) had strengths in psychomotor and technical skills and in developing therapeutic relationships with clients requiring long-term care, and (4) needed further knowledge in the area of the psychosocial needs of clients with chronic illness.

Jacob created a learning plan that acknowledged his existing strengths and focused on those "hard" and "soft" skills needed to work effectively with chronically ill clients requiring long-term care.

Through his environmental scan, Jacob identified broad trends and needs related to care of the adult client with chronic illness and of long-term clients in general. On the basis of information from his scan and self-assessment, he decided to request an adult in-patient medical placement for the first term and an outpatient clinic targeting adult clients at various phases of chronic illness for his final term.

Data from your career vision, environmental scan, and self-assessment help you interpret and structure your learning experiences in a way that is relevant and meaningful to you. The more you learn and reflect on your development as a nurse, the more you can begin to influence your learning experiences.

In most nursing educational programs, students are required to complete their nursing practice placements in organizations that provide experiences congruent with the general goals of the curriculum. Knowing the competencies necessary to achieve expertise in your area of interest can help you make the best of any practice placement experience, even if the placement is not of your choosing. Your career vision, together with a comprehensive scan of the environment and data from your self-assessment, will provide you with the information you need to capitalize on available learning opportunities.

In the previous example, Jacob's awareness of his values, interests, knowledge, and areas for further development provided a direction for his professional educational goals that he could use to guide his learning in any setting. By formulating a learning plan focused on skill development for the care of long-term clients, he could shape his nursing practice learning experience to enhance his skills in working with clients experiencing chronic illness, even if his nursing practice placement was primarily in acute care. Alternatively, he could focus on those skills that are transferable between acute care and chronic care.

Another fourth-year nursing student described how information from the self-assessment process helped him evaluate different nursing practice experiences:

> Throughout my 4 years, I would imagine "putting on the hat" of a specialty of nursing that had caught my attention, and I would create a career vision for each "hat." I would gather information about this particular area through reading, talking to nurses, and attending conferences. I was assessing the match between my interests and talents (gathered through the self-assessment) and the nursing specialty that interested me at that time.

Through ongoing self-assessment, this student recognized his strength in interpersonal communication, specifically in the establishment of therapeutic goal-directed relationships with individual clients. He also valued the mutuality of the nurse–client relationship. This self-knowledge helped him evaluate the fit between an area of nursing practice and a unique professional skill:

> I became interested in nursing informatics and had a related career vision. I went to conferences, read books, and talked to some nurses in the informatics area. I imagined the work I would be doing and explored what I would need to get involved. In the end, it didn't feel right to me. I liked computers and had a good idea of their potential in the nursing profession, but I wanted to work more with people and ideas, not with

machines, data, and policy. My interest in informatics as a career focus faded and was replaced by a new interest—a new "hat" and a vision that was more congruent with my values and strengths.

A third-year student found that by keeping her values at the centre of her nursing practice placement planning, she was able to develop competencies and expertise that would be an asset in any setting:

My mother had to spend a fair amount of time in the hospital, and I was so appreciative of the nurses who took the time to talk to us and help us, as her family, understand what was happening and how we could help her. I don't know what specialty I want to work in, but my vision is that I practise family-centred care. I am known for my expertise in communicating not only with clients but also with families and health care colleagues. Knowing this, I make a point to have the development of competencies related to family-centred care and communication as my learning goal for each placement. If I let my instructor and the other nurses on the unit know about my interest in these areas, they can assign me to clients who will offer the opportunity to work on these professional competencies.

Now you are ready to complete your self-assessment in Activity 3.

Activity (3) Completing Your Self-Assessment

With your vision and your environmental scan in mind, consider the following questions. They can help you understand who you are and what is important to you. Your answers will give you the words to describe your unique self, what you like to do, and what you have to offer. As you start to document your answers, you can begin to write your own story. Your story should include all the important personal and professional events in your life and how they relate to one another.

1. VALUES: WHAT ARE MY PRIORITIES?

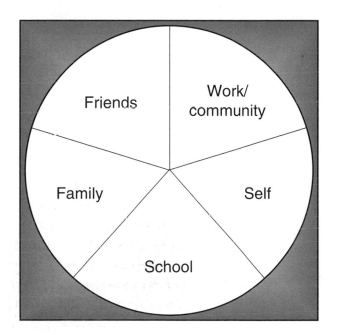

Mark the percentage of time you spend daily in each section of the circle. Now ask yourself the following questions:

➤ What is most important to me in my current nursing education experiences?
Examples: access to professional role models, a good fit between coursework and nursing practice experiences, opportunity to spend time with clients, program responsiveness to current health care realities, respectful relationships with teachers and student colleagues, acceptance of differences, accessible and approachable faculty members

➤ What is important to me as a nursing student and in my personal life?
Examples: relationships, fairness, honesty, balance, knowing my strengths and limitations

➤ What are my key values?

➤ Who or what are the significant persons or things in my life that I need to consider at this time?
Examples: spending time with family, spouse or partner, boyfriend or girlfriend; part-time job

2. KNOWLEDGE AND SKILLS

➤ What knowledge and skills have I developed both personally and professionally in my nursing program and outside of my nursing educational experiences?
Examples: self-directed learning, resourcefulness, flexibility, therapeutic communication [empathy, support, listening]

➤ What new knowledge and skills have I acquired since my last self-assessment?
Examples: technical skills in medical-surgical areas [such as IV monitoring, complex dressings, medication administration]; leadership skills in delivering reports and in participating in interdisciplinary case meetings

➢ What are my strengths?
Examples: communication skills [specifically empathy, open-ended questions, and establishing positive rapport]; organizational skills; responsibility and accountability in practice; resourcefulness, eagerness, enthusiasm

➢ What are my areas for focused professional development?
Examples: knowledge base regarding the psychosocial care of the client with a chronic illness, confidence in challenging physicians when I need to advocate for a client, documentation skills

➢ What knowledge and skills would I like to develop in my current or next term?
Examples: theory related to coping with chronic illness, family-centred care theory in a community care context, effective client teaching, legal and ethical issues related to outpatient care

➢ What is my preferred learning style?
  Examples: visual; auditory; tactile, kinesthetic, and verbal

If you are not aware of various learning styles, you can simply search "Google" using the term "learning styles," for an introduction to the various types of learning styles. With this introductory information in mind, you can further explore the literature related to learning styles should you require further guidance in describing your values.

3. INTERESTS

➢ What were my interests prior to my entering my nursing program?

➢ What have I liked about my nursing practice placement experience or experiences?
  Examples: developing therapeutic relationships with clients, professional role modelling, positive teamwork

➢ What nursing practice experience has been most exciting for me, and why?
Examples: rehabilitation in which I was able to spend time getting to know clients; a slower pace when I felt I had more control and independence in how I organized my care; time to consult and collaborate with other nurses

➢ What courses have been of most interest to me?
Examples: nursing concepts, psychology, transcultural nursing, community nursing

➢ What placements and courses have I disliked?
Examples: I liked them all because I learned something in each one. The ones that were very fast-paced and "technical" were not as rewarding to me although I learned a lot about organization and "hands-on" skills

➢ What energizes or motivates me?
Examples: receiving positive feedback from faculty; hearing—from clients—that I do make a difference; meeting my own goals; relaxing with family and friends; having a good workout

➢ In what type of learning environment (class, clinical practice) do I perform my best?
Example: any environment in which there is interaction and a lot of discussion and in which I feel that what I have to say or contribute is important

➢ What do I like to do outside of my academic environment?
Examples: spend time outdoors, read, spend time with the people I care about, exercise

➤ What is important to me in my physical environment?
Examples: being located in a warm climate, being located in a rural or urban setting, being located close to my friends and family, being located away from familiar places and people

4. ACCOMPLISHMENTS

➤ What have been my most significant accomplishments in my nursing education to date? Outside of my education?
Examples: invited to join my school's honour society; elected as student representative on school council; told by my employer that I was an excellent "trainer" for new staff; told by my preceptor that I have very good leadership skills for my level; have a lot of good friends and am a good friend to others

➤ How can I describe those times when I made a difference?
Examples: When I had my placement at the rehabilitation unit, I organized a game show for the residents and staff. The staff said they had not seen the residents have so much fun in a long time.

Your Reality Check

A reality check is about seeking feedback regarding your strengths and key areas for development. The reality check can help you broaden your view of yourself because others often see you differently from the way you see yourself. Once you have crafted your career vision, conducted your environmental scan, and answered the question, "Who am I?" it is important to validate your answers by doing a reality check. It will provide information that will help you answer the next critical question, "How do others see me?"

Students often find that the reality check provides an opportunity to be informed or reminded of strengths and attributes that they do not recognize in themselves. Keep in mind that your social, family, and community networks are also important sources of feedback about your knowledge, skills, strengths, and limitations. Armed with your vision and with regular formal evaluations from faculty, peers, and nursing contacts, as well as with your expanding nursing experience and your initial assessment of your accomplishments as you enter nursing, you have what you need to update your self-assessment on an ongoing basis.

Why Is a Reality Check Crucial?

Feedback affirms where we shine and sometimes identifies knowledge or skill gaps that need to be filled. As a student, you receive and respond to feedback on a continual basis. A good deal of the feedback you receive is tied to specific course or curriculum goals. Although this feedback is of value in determining and reinforcing your expanding professional strengths and areas for further development, it may not address the areas of self-assessment that you would like confirmed or viewed from another perspective. Therefore, be prepared to request specific feedback related to your self-assessment if your course and program feedback does not address all your unique needs.

How Do You Do a Reality Check?

Start with those individuals you trust—family, student peers, your mentor, and others who know you well. Then consider getting feedback from an individual that you know not too well (perhaps a preceptor or another nurse in your nursing practice placement area), and ask him or her the same questions. You can also refer to your practice placement evaluations and course feedback. The reality check component of the self-assessment process can strengthen your confidence in communicating your skills and uniqueness to colleagues, potential employers, and other professionals. For example, during the reality check step, a third-year nursing student became aware of a strength she had not previously identified:

"I took my career vision and self-assessment to a faculty member that I really like and respect. She confirmed the strengths that I had identified and, to my surprise, added something that I never would have considered. She said my sense of humour was excellent and that it allowed me to establish rapport with clients in a very gentle and non-threatening manner. Now when I care for clients, I am conscious of my use of humour and can see that it is unique and can be therapeutic. She also connected me with others who do the kind of work that I hope to do in the future."

Now you are ready to do your reality check. Complete Activity 4.

Activity ④ Reality Check

> **R**eview your career vision and self-assessment, and re-read your accomplishments. Then, ask yourself the following questions.

➤ What feedback have I received from faculty members, preceptors, mentor, clients, student colleagues, friends, and family regarding my achievements?

➤ What did they identify as my strengths and key areas for development?

➤ What three adjectives would they (or did they) use to describe me, both within and outside the academic or nursing practice environment or workplace? Why?

➢ How did my assessment of my accomplishments compare with others' assessments?

➢ What has changed since my last reality check?

Piece together all the data, and create a written summary of your strengths and challenges. With an accurate sense of who you are and how others see you, you will be ready to explore a range of opportunities and determine how you can focus your next learning experience.

What Have You Accomplished?

You have put your dream into words. The environmental scan gave you valuable information to consider and use to understand nursing issues, trends, and resources across a number of levels, focusing on your career vision. Your self-assessment has allowed you to think about what is important to you, what you do well, and what you need to learn and develop further so that you can progress toward your career vision. Together, your vision, scan, and self-assessment help you get a sense of the fit and gaps between where you are now and where you wish to be in the future.

What Is Your Next Step?

Action! The next step of the career planning process guides you in making plans to use your educational program to determine what you need to learn to move toward your career vision. You know what is around you, you know yourself, and you have your dream. Go for it!

DEVELOPING YOUR STRATEGIC CAREER PLAN

What Are Career Plans?

Career plans are like the learning plans you may be asked to develop throughout your academic career. In fact, as you advance in your education, your learning plan should be your career plan. Whether you view your learning plan and your career plan as one plan or as two separate plans, your career plan will guide you in working with your educational supports and resources to achieve your career goals.

A strategic career plan is a blueprint for action. You are now ready to specify the goals, activities, timelines, and resources you need to achieve your career vision. In this part of the process, you start to put on paper the specific strategies you will use to take charge of your future. The strategic career plan is always a work-in-progress, the object of continual evaluation. As a student, you will be constantly revisiting your vision, scanning your environment, assessing yourself, receiving feedback from others, and evaluating and re-evaluating your goals and your plans for reaching them.

Why Should I Develop a Career Plan?

Having a strategic plan helps you take advantage of each planned or unanticipated learning experience. Whatever your career vision and specific career goals, a plan will allow you to recognize unexpected or "accidental" learning experiences as opportunities and, ultimately, to take control of a rewarding career.

The key to a good plan is to ensure that it is both uniquely yours and easily converted into action within your educational experience. It must be derived from your career vision and outline specific actions that you can take to achieve clearly defined goals. Having a strategic career plan helps you make the career goals that are related to your career vision action oriented. You may have more than one strategic career plan at the same time, as stated by one student:

> In such turbulent times, I feel that I must have several backup plans ready to go at once. I keep my career vision true to my values and interests but fairly broad because I must be ready to shift my specific career goals or options at the drop of a hat. This flexibility and multiple career options allow me to sleep at night, knowing that if I don't get a particular job, I have lots of other possibilities that are still in keeping with my career vision.

How Should I Plan?

A strategic career plan includes identification of the following:

✦ Goals
✦ Action steps
✦ Resources
✦ Timelines
✦ Indicators of success

Document your plan—in writing! The exercise of "writing it down" forces you to include each of the critical components and makes it easier for you to continually review, refine, evaluate, and re-evaluate both your goals and your progress. It also helps you make a commitment to yourself to work on making your plan become reality.

Set Goals

With your career vision, environmental scan, and self-assessment completed, set your short-term and long-term career goals, or your vision will remain only a dream. Choosing and setting goals means that you are serious about taking charge of your learning. When choosing your career goals, always ask yourself, "What do I hope to achieve by pursuing this goal?" Remember to keep the goals specific, time framed, reachable, and relevant. Will anyone who reads them understand what you are trying to accomplish? Do you have actual target dates for achievement? Are your goals realistic enough to be attainable? Are the goals in tune with your future needs?

Career goals should be realistic (I can do it), desirable (I want to do it), and motivating (I will work to make it happen). Remember that you will re-evaluate and alter your career goals as you move toward your career vision, or you may perhaps change your vision as you encounter new experiences in your educational program. Even if you change your vision, you can build on the activities and resources you have used in meeting previous goals.

DAGMAR

To begin a strategic career plan, Dagmar, a fourth-year student with a career vision of being an advanced practice nurse in neonatal intensive care, developed the following goals:

Career Vision: I am an expert advanced-practice nurse in an active neonatal intensive care unit (NICU) in a large urban teaching hospital. I work with an interdisciplinary team to provide a high quality of family-centred care to premature infants and their families. I feel confident in providing a high level of care to neonates and am perceived by my colleagues to have expertise in family-centred care practices. I serve as a preceptor to senior-level students completing their nursing practice placement in the NICU. My contributions are valued, and in return, I demonstrate my respect for the contributions of others. My organization supports both formal and informal professional development philosophically and financially. I enjoy going to work each day.

Career Goal for Academic Year: At the end of the fourth year of my nursing program, I will have the necessary competencies to be considered for an entry-level position in an NICU.

Short-Term Goals:
1. Use nursing practice placement experiences in fourth year to develop competencies in this area of practice
2. Find a mentor in the School of Nursing with expertise in advanced practice nursing and pediatrics
3. Network with other nurses in the NICU through a professional organization and related interest groups.

Long-Term Goal: Get a staff nurse position in an NICU on graduation.

Specify the Action Steps

Once you have determined your goals, use specific action steps to further break down goals into discrete and concrete activities. Action steps complete the sentence, "In order to achieve this goal, I will . . . ."

DAGMAR Dagmar chose the following action steps to achieve her short-term goals:

1. Through my environmental scan, identify the overall professional skills and specific nursing practice competencies that are most important to working and functioning competently in an NICU
2. Update my self-assessment with these competencies in mind
3. Meet with the nursing practice placement coordinator to discuss placement experiences for fourth year that will help me develop competencies in this area
4. Talk to up to three faculty members who could possibly be mentors in advanced practice nursing, neonatal intensive care, pediatrics, or all three areas
5. Find the names of senior students and program alumni who have experienced a nursing practice placement (or currently work) in an NICU

Identify Resources

Having identified specific action steps to take, you are now ready to look at the resources you may need to achieve your goal. The process of developing a plan requires you to think about who and what will help you implement your plan. Making a thoughtful inventory of your available and potential resources is the first step you should take to begin to implement the action steps associated with each of your goals.

DAGMAR To achieve her goals, Dagmar identified as resources the school nursing practice placement coordinator; faculty members with an interest in pediatrics, neonatal intensive care, or both; the nursing student association representative in her school of nursing; the student interest group of her professional nursing organization; her nursing practice advisor; her preceptor from her last nursing practice placement; and a potential mentor.

Once you have determined the resources you will require, you will be ready to set timelines to accomplish your action steps.

Establish Timelines

If your goal is personally motivating and your plan is realistic and concrete, assigning timelines ensures that you allocate your resources in an efficient and ultimately rewarding way. Timelines should suit your particular needs and fit your personal priorities. In the previous example, Dagmar realized she would need to achieve most of her action plans before the end of the school term. She gave herself 5 weeks to achieve all of her action plans, and she scheduled one to two specific action steps per week.

Timelines can be modified, but including them at the outset is critical to developing an effective career plan.

Identify the Indicators of Success

How will you know that your plan is working? If you have documented your plan (including specific action steps, required resources, and timelines), you have a good start at identifying indicators of success. Think about what you are hoping to accomplish with your plan. For Dagmar, identifying the indicators of success involved having a list of both "hard" and "soft" skills necessary to be a competent NICU nurse, revising her self-assessment, meeting with the placement coordinator and the student nursing association representative, finding out when the next professional association student interest group meeting would be held, and making appointments with the three faculty members who were active in pediatrics and in the NICU.

As you design your own plan, think about what success would look like for you. Career plans should be dynamic, responsive to personal circumstances, and professionally stimulating. You should be ready to adjust your plan as aspects of your vision or self-assessment change, as your continually updated environmental scan indicates that significant changes have occurred around you, and as you move forward in your education.

Now you are ready to develop your own strategic career plan. Complete Activity 5.

Activity ⑤ Developing Your Strategic Career Plan

A well-developed strategic plan not only helps you realize your career vision but also enables you to recognize and take advantage of other career opportunities as they occur.

✦ Start by putting your written career vision right in front of you.

✦ Identify your short-term and long-term career goals.

✦ Complete the following strategic career plan outline.

STRATEGIC CAREER PLAN

Career Vision:

Career Goals:

Action Steps	Resources	When to Accomplish	How Will I Know I Have Succeeded?

Thinking of Graduate Studies?

Pursuing graduate studies may have been your intent from the beginning of your nursing education, or it may be a more recent decision arising from your career vision.

As with any other career decision, you have some important choices to make. Many students ask the following questions:

+ How do I choose the right graduate program?
+ How do I sort out the benefits of one program or university compared with another?
+ What types of questions should I be asking?
+ What can I be doing in my undergraduate program to position me for success in both application process and program of study?

You can use your strategic career plan to help you answer these important questions and also integrate it into your existing career planning work (that is, into every phase), or you might actually do a parallel career planning exercise devoted specifically to the pursuit of graduate studies. Either way, you can begin by expanding your environmental scan to include the nature and role of graduate programs in nursing or in related disciplines. Gather information related to the types of available programs and how they advance the careers of nurses in your area of interest. You can also learn about general graduate education entry requirements (i.e., those that are usually required regardless of the university or program). With the information from your scan in mind, return to your self-assessment and focus on identifying gaps and strengths most relevant to this career planning strategy. For example, because grades and grade point average or class standing are almost always a key issue in graduate applications, review your grades and (if necessary) consider how you can ensure that you meet the general requirements.

The next step in the development of your strategic career plan for graduate studies can focus on gathering information related to the types of programs offered and mode of delivery (online, campus-based, or a mix or hybrid of online and campus-based), faculty resources, flexibility of programs with respect to full-time and part-time study options, access to online courses, timelines for degree completion, and career opportunities during and on completion of the program. Remember to ask for the philosophy and mission statement of the program so you can determine whether the stated values and beliefs about teaching and learning are a good fit with the values you have identified in your self-assessment. Reviewing the profiles of faculty members at the schools of interest is another way to see whether the program has a faculty with expertise in your fields of interest. You can also arrange to meet with resource persons within the faculty and with alumni or current students in the program to discuss your questions. Do not forget that with each contact you are marketing yourself at the same time you are seeking information. The next section of this guide (Phase Five of the Model) offers specific marketing tips and strategies.

Use your self-knowledge and your career vision to assess congruency among your values, interests, learning style, career goals, and the various graduate programs. You can then more accurately assess how well any program will help you progress toward your career vision. This is where knowing theoretical biases and approaches to teaching and learning, among other program characteristics, can help you make a decision that is a good fit with who you are, how you learn, and what is important to you. At any stage during this process, it can be helpful to seek the perspective of your mentor, student colleagues, and significant other. It can also be beneficial to speak with students you know who are currently engaged in a graduate program or who are recent graduates. Informal sources of information and guidance are often valuable resources as you prepare for your graduate education.

As you can see, using your strategic career plan to prepare for graduate studies prompts you to revisit all stages of the Career Planning and Development Model with a specific focus in mind. The work you will do as you explore graduate studies illustrates the dynamic nature of the career planning and development process and how it guides you in your efforts to achieve your career dreams.

What Have You Accomplished?

You have a game plan! You have used your vision, your environmental scan, and your self-assessment to develop some plans that you can begin to implement now. You have a concrete place to start. Your vision is on its way to becoming a reality.

What Is Your Next Step?

It is time to start telling others what you have just confirmed for yourself. You have a vision; you know your current strengths, values, interests, and accomplishments; you know how they fit with the world of nursing; and you have a plan. Now you need to share all of this with the people who can help you.

MARKETING YOURSELF

Student Nurses as Self-Marketers

Marketing simply means being able to communicate confidently and effectively to others your vision, strengths, interests, and goals, as well as the contributions you can make to professional practice. What better place is there than your nursing education to acquire self-marketing skills?

A third-year student made the following comments about self-marketing:

> Although I was already aware of the importance of developing a career plan, I learned that the process does not end there; rather, the plan needs to be put into action through the use of various self-marketing

strategies. I want to make sure I get the job that is right for me. For this reason, I feel it is important to implement appropriate self-marketing strategies so I can represent myself in the best possible way.

The key to successful marketing is to develop an approach that is congruent with your values and communication style and true to your abilities. When you completed your self-assessment, you identified your values and beliefs and evaluated your expanding nursing experience, accomplishments, strengths, and areas for improvement. Now that you have taken a close look at the things that make you unique, you can most effectively promote yourself and meet your goals by making and keeping yourself visible. Your strengths, coupled with a commitment and a belief in yourself, make you your own best marketer.

Why Marketing Yourself Is Important

Intentionally or unintentionally, you market who and what you are in every professional encounter. During each nursing practice placement experience, each involvement in the classroom environment, and each meeting with a faculty member or student colleague, you communicate (directly or indirectly) your values and your professional identity. Thoughtful and intentional self-marketing enables you to take control of how you represent yourself to others. In this section, you will learn about the resources and tools that form the foundation of an effective self-marketing strategy; you can then use this strategy to create your own opportunities.

It is important to keep in mind that when you are actively marketing through your résumé and interview processes, employers may refer to Web sites such as Facebook, blogs, and Myspace to learn more about you as a potential employee. Go to Google (http://www.google.ca/) and search your name to find out what personal information about you is accessible to potential employers and the general public. Consider the type of information, graphics, and photographs you offer through these sites when you are endeavouring to market your professional attributes.

How Can I Market Myself?

For student nurses, self-marketing is facilitated by establishing a network, acquiring a mentor, and developing written and verbal communication skills.

Networking and Establishing Support Groups

Establishing a network is a fundamental step in self-marketing. Networking can serve many purposes for nursing students. It involves meeting with a variety of people who share similar interests, who practise in areas of nursing that are attractive to you, and who can offer new ideas, perspectives, and opportunities. Besides being a valuable way to establish and maintain your sense of professional identity, networking also offers the opportunity to inform others of your interests, activities, and hopes for your future practice.

Networking can produce significant results if you believe in yourself and are committed and prepared to work at it. Be mindful that your networking activities will likely become more focused as you progress in your educational program. Initially, you may feel unsure about the most appropriate place to start to network. In the early years of your program, it may be most beneficial to concentrate your networking activities within your school of nursing. As you start to develop some questions and focus related to your career vision, you can benefit from networking resources in the broader nursing community.

Throughout your nursing education, but particularly in its early stages, it is important to discover who your classmates are and how you can establish a sense of involvement in your school of nursing. Meeting students at all levels of your program will help you find others with similar goals and interests. It will also offer you the chance to find out about interesting courses, nursing practice placements, and resources, not to mention the support that you can enjoy through your interactions with others who are experiencing similar challenges and adjustments. Becoming actively involved with professional student groups is an excellent way to meet student colleagues and provides many advantages, including the following:

✦ The opportunity to meet and work with a large number of faculty members
✦ Support in attending conferences and workshops locally, provincially, and nationally
✦ Opportunities to gain experience in working on committees and in public speaking
✦ The development of overall leadership skills

The first step in developing your own network is to make a list of people you think may be helpful to you. Consider all the facets of your life—social, family, school, and work—as you identify potentially helpful people. In addition to student associations, faculty members represent another opportunity for networking that is at your fingertips. Each faculty member has recognized expertise in one or more areas of clinical nursing practice, research, and education. The exchange of interests and ideas can be mutually rewarding for you and the faculty member.

The process of networking with your classmates can be both formal and informal. Joining student groups and committees is one formal means of meeting and working with fellow students. A fourth-year student described the following experience:

> I became active with student groups within 2 months of starting nursing school. From there, things just blossomed until I was making connections with students on a national level through my professional nursing students association. Now that I am ready to graduate and look for a job, I have a network of colleagues I can call on for advice and direction.

Involvement with the student nurses association allowed this student to meet others both from her nursing program and from other nursing schools. The many advantages associated with becoming involved with formal student groups in the academic setting include (1) the opportunity to meet and work with a large number of faculty members; (2) support in attending provincial (or state), national, and even international conferences and workshops; (3) opportunities to gain experience in working on committees and in public speaking; and (4) the development of overall leadership skills. Whether you choose formal or informal settings or both, such involvement means networking with your peers; sharing your vision, goals, and interests with them; and allowing them to keep you in mind during their experiences. You, in turn, can do the same for them as you encounter new experiences.

The exchange of ideas can be a mutually rewarding experience for you and the faculty member. One student reported the following networking experiences in a school of nursing:

> In my final year, I volunteered to be my class representative for student council and also became a member of my school's nursing honour society steering committee. These opportunities allowed me to learn more about faculty members and to interact differently with them from the way I would if we were discussing a test grade or paper. The faculty offered guidance, resources, and support.

Another excellent opportunity for networking is provided by volunteer activities. The people you meet while volunteering will help expand your network. Volunteer work is an opportunity to develop new skills and gain experience and insight into a new environment. A good place to start is in your school of nursing. Many faculty and fellow students are involved in committees and organizations and would welcome new ideas, energy, and enthusiasm. Your career vision can also help you identify volunteer activities. For example, if you are interested in working with clients in palliative care, you may consider volunteering on a palliative care unit. The time commitment required for volunteer activities varies, so you need to check whether you can fit outside volunteer activities into your academic schedule without putting undue stress on yourself.

Once you have established your network (or networks), you can target certain individuals and begin to build and maintain a support group. Your support group can consist of fellow students and faculty members who believe in you and want to see you succeed. Surround yourself with individuals who keep a positive attitude and are a source of confidence as you develop an action plan to reach your career goals and, ultimately, your career vision. Seek out those whose feedback you value and whose emotional support you can count on, particularly when you take risks.

You may want to build your support group right now. As you engage in the career planning process, a support group of your peers can help you explore your options and problem-solve as you work with the Model—and network!

Finding a Mentor

The second step in your self-marketing strategy should be to acquire a mentor. A mentor is someone who takes personal and professional interest in your career development. Your mentor should be someone with more experience and wisdom who supports and encourages you as you grow and develop in your career (Donner & Wheeler, 2007). Your mentor will guide and support you through all areas of the career planning and development process as you transform your dreams into reality. In the nursing world, mentors generally are experienced nurses who know the ins and outs of the health care environment, have more connections, and have more access to information than less experienced and often younger nurses have. Do not restrict yourself to the nursing community when finding a mentor. Your social and community connections are also excellent resources.

Determine the type of mentor you need and where to find one by reflecting on your career vision and looking at your self-assessment to help you identify exactly the type of help and support you require. Desirable characteristics of any mentor include patience, enthusiasm, knowledge, a sense of humour, and respect (Donner & Wheeler, 2007). Other important considerations when you are determining the fit between you and a potential mentor are the ability of the mentor to be available to you in terms of supporting you to achieve your career goals, the potential mentor's leadership and teaching style, and the willingness of the mentor to commit to the mentoring relationship. This commitment must also be shared by you as the "mentee."

Through coaching and moral support, your mentor can help you scan the environment and can give feedback as you assess your own strengths, identify your career goals, and develop a career plan that fits with your vision. Your mentor can also help you develop your skills in marketing and open doors that will enable you to meet others who can support your career goals and activities (Donner & Wheeler, 2007). Of course, not everyone needs or wants a mentor. However, having a mentor is one of the valuable ways to ensure your career success—so consider it.

A mentor may be a faculty member who has taken a special interest in you, has influenced your career decisions, and has helped open doors for you. You may also encounter nurses in your nursing practice placement experiences, summer employment, volunteer activities, and other professional activities who are role models for you. Once you have identified a possible mentor, create both informal and formal opportunities for you to get to know each other. Such opportunities include volunteer work on similar projects or choosing to sit on a committee of which the mentor is a member.

A fourth-year student described his relationship with a mentor as follows:

> My nursing practice advisor from third year has become an excellent mentor. We have had numerous opportunities to work together, and she has a good idea of my career vision, my strengths, and key areas for my ongoing development. She has provided me with advice and support regarding my career direction, and she has suggested other individuals I could meet with to discuss my interests. I feel that working with a mentor is a great self-marketing strategy that I can continue to use long after I graduate.

Another student described her mentor in the following way:

> She was an influential faculty member who took the time to help me and get to know me. She listened to my vision, identified opportunities for growth, and encouraged me to explore them. She provided opportunities for me to be involved both within the school and in the broader nursing community. I learned from her professional presentation, and she seemed to take extra time to help me with my professional development.

A senior student thus described her experience in asking a faculty member to be her mentor:

> I really enjoyed the nursing practice instructor I had in my medical-surgical placement in the second year of my program. Even in her role as an instructor, she really seemed to make a difference to the clients. She also got along well with the staff and was involved in a lot of professional activities. I often thought that I would like to be just like her when I got to be a "real" nurse! I never told her that I admired her; I just assumed she would know that. In my fourth year, she was my nursing practice advisor for my final placement. She was still as active and as impressive as I remembered her to be. I decided to tell her that I considered her to be a great professional role model. I also asked her if she would be my mentor. To my surprise, she said that she would be honoured to act as my mentor, and since that meeting, she has met with me to go over my career vision and self-assessment and has already begun to inform me of activities and people she thinks would be helpful to my career.

Developing Your Communication Skills: Marketing Yourself on Paper

Creating a targeted résumé and other written communication (e.g., business cards) is an important part of self-marketing.

Résumés. Your résumé is one of your most valuable written self-marketing strategies. It is a summary of your skills and accomplishments. A résumé is also a way to monitor your progress in building the strengths and expertise that you have identified in your self-assessment.

Creating a résumé requires preparation, patience, practice, practice, and practice! Remember, there is no such thing as a "one size fits all" résumé. You must customize your résumé to ensure that it is effective for each specific opportunity you are pursuing. Use your résumé as a strategic marketing tool to accentuate the accomplishments, skills, and knowledge you identified as part of your self-assessment. It is an essential part of many nursing practice placements as well as the job search process. You will need to collect some data about a potential placement or job opportunity before you can customize your résumé. Learn about the organization and the role of students in the organization and in the specific unit, and scan the environment to determine available learning opportunities and how your learning goals may fit with those opportunities.

It is helpful to have a "junk drawer" résumé where you can document all your nursing practice experiences (with a brief description of the skills and accomplishments resulting from each experience), nursing and non-nursing jobs, volunteer activities, extracurricular professional development activities, and professionally related qualifications. Create headings for all categories of activities (i.e., education, awards, nursing practice experiences, professional activities, professional memberships, employment history, and volunteer activities). If you find that you have headings but no activities to place under them, then you know that one of your career development activities should be related to that area of your professional life. When it is time to submit a résumé for a nursing practice placement application or for a job, you can create a customized résumé by selecting the information from your "junk drawer" version that is most relevant to the placement or job for which you are applying.

A student résumé has three unique aspects: (1) the list of selected nursing practice placements; (2) the nursing practice experience summary and outcome competencies and accomplishments; and (3) the documentation of past working experiences, including summer and part-time employment. The list of selected nursing practice placements includes those placement experiences through which you developed and enhanced nursing practice competencies and the knowledge most relevant to the job for which you are applying. Limit the list of selected placements to two or three experiences, with the description of responsibilities, accomplishments, and competencies focused on those that relate directly to the advertised nursing role. The nursing practice experience summary informs the employer of the scope of practice experiences you have had during your nursing career. These experiences can simply be listed; include those completed in the early years of your nursing program and those that provided you with fundamental nursing knowledge and skills.

The components of a student résumé are illustrated in Appendix A. You may also download a résumé exercise and résumé template from http://www.elsevier.ca/ DonnerWheeler/ to begin building your résumé-writing skills.

Your résumé should always be accompanied by a one-page cover letter. The purpose of a cover letter is to encourage the recipient to read your résumé more carefully to determine how your specific learning goals, experience, and abilities fit with his or her organization or society. It should be printed out on personal letterhead paper and attached to your personal business card; together, these will provide all the details the reader needs to get in touch with you. An example of a cover letter can be found in Appendix B.

Electronic Résumés. Bookey-Bassett (2004) notes the significant impact that technology has had on the job search process. Many employers now prefer to receive résumés by e-mail. Electronic résumés can be sent as a Microsoft Word attachment, in a Web portfolio, or on a compact disc (CD) (Bookey-Bassett, 2004; Dixson, 2001; Smith, 1999). Using career portfolios or CD résumés or portfolios allows you to creatively convey your competencies and accomplishments with multimedia technology. Resources for developing electronic résumés can be found in the "Career Planning and Development Resources" section at the end of this guide.

If the employer specifically requests an electronic résumé, determine if they require one particular format. Copy and paste the résumé into the body of a test e-mail message and send it back to yourself (or to a friend who uses a different e-mail program) to see how the recipient will view your résumé. Keep in mind that when you are applying for a job electronically, a cover letter should accompany your résumé. The letter should be sent in the text portion; send the résumé as an attachment to the e-mail message.

Business Cards. Business cards provide a simple and professional way to introduce yourself to others and to ensure that they do not forget you. Student business cards need have only your name, phone number, and e-mail address. As one student observed:

> I never thought it would be appropriate for students to carry and distribute their own business cards. After a career planning and development workshop, I went home and designed one with a computer program I have. I think this strategy is an effective and creative means of giving others a way to reach me by telephone, fax, or e-mail. I included only my name, the fact that I was a student nurse, my university, and contact information. I was encouraged to keep the card simple, and it looks great. Having my own business card also makes me feel more professional and important.

Another student shared the following:

> Having my own business card makes me feel professional, valued, and significant. I remember when I handed my first business card to a colleague of mine in class. She was very impressed by the professionalism it conveyed. Distributing your own business card not only conveys professionalism but puts the "finishing touch" to the end of an encounter. When done correctly, I think it makes the perfect first and last impression.

Developing Your Communication Skills: Marketing Yourself in Person

Each time you meet someone new, you are presented with a marketing opportunity to accentuate your positives, take credit for your accomplishments, share your professional goals, and remind others of what you have to contribute. To seize these opportunities effectively, you should rehearse a short self-promotional statement. Then when you meet people and are asked to talk about yourself, you will be ready to clearly, concisely, and confidently articulate your career vision, your current level of knowledge and skills, your present and future career goals, and your unique contributions. You do not need to wait for people to come to you. Become active in your school, student and professional associations, and interest groups, and contribute to an initiative that will help you both build and profile your talents and accomplishments.

The Interview. The interview provides another excellent self-marketing opportunity. You will need finely honed interview skills whether you are interviewed for a nursing practice placement, a job, graduate school, or a volunteer position and whether you are interviewed by a professional association or by a community agency. An interview is a powerful self-marketing opportunity to present your interests, knowledge, skills, and potential in the most positive and appropriate manner.

Many nursing practice placement agencies now require that students participate in an interview before being considered for a nursing practice placement. You should plan for these interviews as thoughtfully and thoroughly as you would for a job interview. If your career vision, self-assessment, and strategic career plan are up to date and if you have done your preparation, your chances of having a successful interview are good. At the interview, it is important to have clear learning goals based on your self-assessment, nursing program objectives, and knowledge of the nursing practice setting.

Your answers to the interview questions can demonstrate that you have relevant interests, entry skills, knowledge, and (most importantly) the enthusiasm and ability to learn and make contributions to the placement unit. The interview also gives you an opportunity to have your questions answered so that if you are offered the position, you can consult with your mentor, nursing practice placement coordinator, or nursing practice advisor to make a well-informed decision about whether the placement is the right one for you.

Some individuals find it helpful to audiotape or videotape themselves in a mock interview so that they can identify their strengths and the areas they would like to improve on prior to experiencing the "real thing." Ask a student colleague to help you with this exercise and offer you some feedback. Your mentor is another excellent resource for practising your interview skills.

JANET In preparation for an interview at a nursing practice placement agency, Janet obtained (1) copies of the philosophy statement of the unit to which she was applying, as well as that of the nursing department; (2) a copy of the hospital's strategic plan and a registered nurse job description for her clinical practice area; and (3) a schedule of selected professional development opportunities she could take advantage of as a student in the nursing practice placement setting. She then spoke with two students who had experience in that unit. Finally, she met with her mentor (a faculty member with expertise in her chosen nursing practice area) to discuss how the skills and accomplishments identified in her self-assessment and her related learning goals would fit with the available learning opportunities and with the philosophies and plans of the nursing practice unit and organization. Janet also participated in a mock interview with her mentor before her nursing practice interview.

See http://www.elsevier.ca/DonnerWheeler/ on the Web for an exercise to help you build your interview skills.

References. Faculty members, mentors, clinical practice preceptors, part-time and summer job employers, and contacts from volunteer activities can be appropriate sources of references for students. It is important that you select as referees individuals who are familiar with your current level of nursing practice skill development and recent practice accomplishments relevant to the practice area to which you are applying. If a referee is not knowledgeable about your recent work, provide him or her with a copy of your résumé and any other information that supports your application for the job (e.g., vision, self-assessment, strategic career plan, nursing practice placement evaluations, or completed clinical practice projects).

It is important to ask potential referees well in advance if they would be willing to provide a positive reference for you. After a job interview, offer the names of your referees if you would like to pursue employment with that organization. Contact your referees each time you give their name as a reference. Inform them of the specific requirements of the job you are seeking, and give them any other information that will help them provide a comprehensive reference. Be sure that your referees have a copy of the résumé you submitted and any new information that may not appear on your résumé.

Self-marketing is about using all your resources to present yourself in the strongest and most positive way. Remember that the most important resource you have for shaping your own future is you! Keep your career vision and goals in mind. Creating an effective self-marketing strategy that works for you takes time, effort, and patience. Following these strategies will contribute to realizing your goals. The following excerpt summarizes Janet's thoughts on the process of career planning:

> Learning about the career planning process motivated me to think more seriously about my career plans and what I have done and need to do to accomplish them. I have realized the need to clarify my plans and put them into action through a number of realistic self-marketing strategies. This experience has allowed me to be more self-directed and actively involved. I believe I have a better understanding of the numerous opportunities available to me and how I can take advantage of them in an effective way.

Complete Activity 6 to assess your marketing readiness.

Activity (6) Marketing Yourself

> **S**elf-marketing is representing yourself in the best way possible by using all your resources.

➤ How is your marketing readiness? Use the following checklist to answer that question:

- ❏ I have a career vision.
- ❏ I know my environment.
- ❏ I know myself.
- ❏ I know I am my best marketer.
- ❏ I know how to network.
- ❏ I have a support group.
- ❏ I have a mentor.
- ❏ I have a current résumé.
- ❏ I have a business card.
- ❏ I have excellent interview skills.

➤ Which areas need some attention? Develop a plan to address those needs.

What I Need To Do	When I Will Do It
1.	1.
2.	2.
3.	3.
4.	4.
5.	5.

What Have You Accomplished?

Congratulations! You have made your first tour through the Career Planning and Development Model. You have learned how you can use your dreams, the environment, self-knowledge, and your career plan to explore how you can influence your educational activities to meet your current and future career goals. You will return to the Model again and again as you build your nursing career. We hope it serves you well!

WHAT NEXT?

Career planning and development is a continuous process—a "work in progress." To ensure that you are getting the most out of your career planning activities, you should consider an overall evaluation of how it is working for you. Complete the following questionnaire after each nursing practice experience and on an annual basis. It will help you determine which phases of the Model need more attention, need updating, or need more consultation and support. You can also use your journal as an ongoing record of how you are moving forward as a student, as a future nurse, and as a person.

How Am I Doing?

Visioning

☐ I can describe my ideal vision for my future.

Scanning

☐ I am aware of the current realities and future trends at the school, local, and national levels within health care and in the nursing profession.

Assessing

☐ I can describe my strengths.

☐ I can describe key areas for development.

☐ I know how others would describe me.

☐ My current academic activities are a good match with my values, beliefs, knowledge, skills, interests, and vision.

Planning

☐ I can identify my career vision and my short- and long-term career goals.

☐ I have a written career development plan in place.

☐ I know what steps to take over the next 3 to 6 months to further my progress toward my career vision.

Marketing

☐ I have established a relevant network.

☐ I have acquired a mentor or am considering acquiring one.

☐ I continue to develop my communication skills.

☐ I have an up-to-date résumé.

3

Choosing Your First Job as a Registered Nurse

Congratulations on successfully completing your nursing program! You have worked hard to achieve your nursing degree. It is a very exciting time to be a nursing graduate. The possibilities are endless, but excitement can be accompanied by anxiety. You have some important decisions to make. Using the Model to guide your exploration and assessment of job opportunities can give you a sense of control and confidence regarding your decision making. Many students ask the following questions:

✦ How can I make sure that I am choosing the job that is right for me?
✦ How can I sort out the benefits of one job offer compared with another?
✦ What types of questions should I be asking?

You are now ready to use the Donner-Wheeler Career Planning and Development Model to help position you to get the job you want. It is important to return to each phase of the Model as you embark on the exciting process of choosing your first position as a registered nurse.

YOUR CAREER VISION

Time to dream again! This is an exciting moment in your personal and professional life. How have you envisioned yourself as a nurse? Use your vision to guide your choice of where to submit your job applications. How do the positions to which you are applying fit with your vision? Can you see the potential of the positions to help you actualize your vision? You have many choices as you move into the current health care system. You are needed and wanted. Your vision can help you make choices that fit with your current interests, needs, knowledge, and dreams.

YOUR ENVIRONMENTAL SCAN

As you prepare to move into the workplace, it is important to update your environmental scan. Include a scan of national, provincial, and local issues and trends. The purpose of this scan is two-fold: (1) to determine the issues and trends in your particular area of interest and focus; and (2) to become aware of the current realities in both the profession and the health care system in general. Knowledge of what is currently happening in your area of interest will help you get a sense of what is "out there" in terms of specific jobs, issues and gaps within those job opportunities, and practice challenges you might be able to anticipate and reflect on as you revisit your self-assessment. Awareness of issues and trends in the profession as well as in the health care system in general will serve you well in the interview process. Your scan could also include enhancing your awareness of general employability skills. The Conference Board of Canada Employability Skills 2000+ list is a list of employability skills that can expand your self-assessment and scanning activities (go to http://www.conferenceboard.ca/education/learning-tools/pdfs/esp2000.pdf and search "Conference Board of Canada Employability Skills" to view the skills list). With this knowledge, you can feel confident responding to potential questions focused on what you see as current and future issues for nurses entering the workforce at this time. The scan can also cue you about questions you might like to ask in an interview.

If you know the agency to which you are applying, a significant focus of your scan should be on learning about the mandate, philosophy, professional practice model, and resources of the nursing department. Obtain a copy of the job description to determine how your skills, knowledge, and interests fit with the job requirements and how to market those qualities. Your scan will also help you determine if the supports, resources, and culture of a given organization fit with your vision and values. It is also important to assess the degree to which organizations acknowledge and respond to the unique challenges experienced by new graduates as they make the transition from students to registered nurses.

YOUR SELF-ASSESSMENT

Return to your self-assessment. This will not be the last time you do a self-assessment, but this is the one time that doing it will serve as a springboard to your first nursing position. Complete this self-assessment with a focus on your values, interests, knowledge, and skills related to your particular career vision. If you do not have one area of interest, complete your assessment with a view to consolidating your overall professional interests, skills, and knowledge base. As you apply for specific jobs, you can refine your assessment to reflect the particular position at hand. In essence, you are streamlining your self-assessment to help you target the position you wish to secure. The position should also allow you to continue to advance toward your career vision. Undoubtedly, the process of completing your assessment will remind you of all that you have learned and of your identity as a unique professional who has much to contribute to nursing.

YOUR STRATEGIC CAREER PLAN

Your strategic career plan can be focused on short-term and long-term goals related to getting the job you want. Your scan has given you important information related to opportunities and realities; your assessment has clarified your current interests, skills, knowledge, and values; and your vision is your future. Using this information as your guide, ask yourself what you need to do to meet your short-term and long-term goals and who can help you. You can focus your activities on getting more information, contacting resources, developing your résumé, or preparing for an interview.

MARKETING

Make an appointment with your mentor to discuss your graduation plans. Bring your mentor up to date with your vision and career-planning activities, and seek specific support to help you assess the relative merits of job opportunities. Your mentor can also assist you as you develop your strategic career plan.

If you would like to seek employment in your current nursing practice placement area, let your preceptor, nursing practice advisor, and nurse manager know of your interest. You have the information from your vision, scan, and self-assessment to effectively market your interest and the contributions you could make as an employee in that setting.

Information from health care agencies can help you determine the fit between your vision, interests, and skills and the goals and philosophies of individual settings. The interview guide in Appendix C outlines the type of information you can seek when preparing for an interview. You can collect this same information long before the interview stage to decide whether you want to consider a particular agency for future employment.

When you select agencies for potential employment, you need to customize your résumé for each employer. Review the résumé and cover letter sections in Chapter 2 as well as Appendix A for tips on résumé development.

You *have* the knowledge you need to select the job that best matches your interests and your vision. You are in the driver's seat; enjoy the ride!

Do You Need More Help?

You have covered a lot of material. If it seems overwhelming or if you are not sure you have a good understanding of it, your first step should be to go back to the beginning of the guide and review the material and activities. Then look at the references provided in the "Career Planning and Development Sources" section at the end of the guide. You can also join or establish a support group with student peers who are also using this guide for their career planning experience. Sharing your questions, ideas, and strategies can provide you with relevant support and new resources. Career resources at your college or university and faculty members with an interest in career development are other supports available to you. The Internet is another valuable resource. You probably already use it a great deal to enhance your nursing education, but consider using it to find resources to help you manage your student career and make sound decisions about your future career. Of course, there are also nursing student and professional organizations that provide many paths to pursue learning and professional growth. You are in a career with numerous and varied opportunities. Yes, there will also be many challenges, but armed with a clear understanding of who you are and what you want to contribute in nursing, you will be ready for that future.

I never lose an opportunity of urging a practical beginning, however small, for it is wonderful how often the mustard-seed germinates and roots itself.

– Florence Nightingale

Samples of Student Résumés

Student Entering Third Year of Baccalaureate Program and Seeking Clinical Placement in a Maternal–Child Setting

Maeve O'Donnell
123 Four Street
City, Province/State Postal/Zip code
Tel: H: (123) 456-7891
E-mail: modonnell@coldmail.com
Fax: (123) 654-9871

Placement Objective: To develop knowledge and professional practice competencies in family-centred care for women during the labour and postpartum experiences.

EDUCATION

Baccalaureate in Nursing
Name of University
City, Province
Anticipated date of completion: May 2005

HONOURS AND AWARDS

Member, University Chapter, Sigma Theta Tau International

SELECTED CLINICAL EXPERIENCES

Nursing Student, 2nd Year, Medical-Surgical Setting
Worked collaboratively within a team nursing model to provide comprehensive care to adults in the postoperative period. Acknowledged for effective communication skills with clients and nursing colleagues, surgery-related client teaching, and leadership skills within scope of student role.

Acquired Competencies: Basic physical assessment skills, aseptic technique, simple and complex dressings, safe medication administration, therapeutic communication skills.

Continued

Nursing Student, 2nd Year, Rehabilitation Medicine

Worked effectively with preceptor in providing comprehensive client care within a primary nursing model. Acknowledged for strong communication skills with older clients, effective psycho-social nursing care, and basic physical care. Contributed to inter-disciplinary client care discussions.

Acquired Competencies: Positive therapeutic communication skills, effective body mechanics, health teaching, family-centred care, discharge planning.

PROFESSIONAL ACTIVITIES

2000–2001	2nd-year representative at School Council
1999–2000	1st-year representative at School Council

PROFESSIONAL MEMBERSHIPS

Student member, Professional Association

EMPLOYMENT HISTORY

1999–
Present

Salesperson, GAP
Part-time position.
Required to work independently, providing supervision and training to new salespersons. Responsible for meeting consumer needs in a professional manner. Utilized effective organizational and management skills. Collaborative member of sales team.

May 2000–
August 2000

Personal Care Assistant, Lakeview Retirement Centre
Summer employment.
Required to work independently, providing basic care to residents. Utilized positive and effective communication skills. Acknowledged for strengths in conveying compassion, sensitivity, and respect to residents and families. Reliable and responsible.

VOLUNTEER ACTIVITIES

May 2000–
Present

Volunteer, Local Hospital Neonatal Unit
Help feed babies 2 hours per week.

Graduating Student Seeking First Nursing Position in a Mental Health Setting

George Donovan
1111 Twelve Street
City, Province/State Postal/Zip code
H (444) 222-3333; W (444) 555-6666
E-mail: donovan@nomail.com
Fax: (444) 777-8888

Career Objective: To secure an entry-level position as a staff nurse in the mental health area, where I can further develop my nursing practice competencies and contribute my growing strengths in therapeutic communication and interdisciplinary teamwork.

EDUCATION

1998–Present   Baccalaureate in Nursing
Name of University
City, Province/State
Anticipated date of completion: May 2003

HONOURS

1999–2000   Dean's List

SELECTED CLINICAL EXPERIENCES

Nursing Student, 4th Year, City Mental Health Outpatient Unit
Young Adult and Adolescent Client Groups.

With preceptor, co-facilitated psychoeducational groups for newly diagnosed young adults and adolescents with schizophrenia. Administered psychotropic medications and monitored the adverse effects of medications. Provided individualized client and family education related to illness and medication.

Acquired Competencies: Administration of Mini-Mental State Examination, with supervision; facilitation of support and psychoeducational groups; individual supportive counselling.

Accomplishments: Developed a medication educational pamphlet targeted at young adults and adolescents.

Nursing Student, 3rd Year,
Community Outreach Program with Focus on Homeless
Provided care to homeless individuals (e.g., foot care, medication administration, shelter arrangements).

Continued

Acquired Competencies: Gained skills in engaging the homeless client, assessing health needs within the context of the individual's lifestyle, and managing issues related to treatment adherence.

Accomplishments: Acknowledged for strengths in developing a positive rapport with hard-to-reach clients and in adapting care to the street setting.

OTHER PLACEMENT EXPERIENCES

2nd year, Rehabilitation Medicine, Surgery, and General Medicine
3rd year, Public Health
4th year, Male Eating Disorders Clinic

PROFESSIONAL ACTIVITIES

2000–2001   Associate Delegate and Official Delegate of the Nursing Students Association

1999–2000   Year representative for School Council

PROFESSIONAL MEMBERSHIPS

Professional Association
Student Interest Group
Mental Health Interest Group

EMPLOYMENT HISTORY

1998–2001   **Health Care Aide**
Summer Employment, Long-term care facility, City
Provided comprehensive care to mentally handicapped clients in a medical centre. Responsible for direct daily care for five clients.

Accomplishments: Organized a family support picnic for residents and families.

1996–1998   **Waiter**
Restaurant, City

Developed skills in organization, time management, and consumer-focused service.

Provided competent and professional service to restaurant patrons. Reliable and responsible.

VOLUNTEER ACTIVITIES

2001–2002   Continue to organize annual family support picnics for residents of a long-term care facility and their families.

9999 90th Ave.
City, Province/State
Postal/Zip Code
Phone Number

Date

Ms. Jane Smith
Program Director
Mental Health Unit
Metropolitan Health Centre
Any City, Province/State, Postal/Zip Code

Dear Ms. Smith:

I am writing in response to the advertisement posted on the Human Resources Bulletin Board for the staff nurse position in the Mental Health Program.

I will be graduating from my nursing baccalaureate program in May 2009. Over the course of my education, I have endeavoured to develop a wide range of professional practice competencies relevant to mental health nursing. I have taken advantage of many learning opportunities, with the goal of achieving strengths in therapeutic communication, psychosocial and mental health assessment and intervention, and interdisciplinary teamwork. I believe I have been successful in obtaining a solid foundation for mental health nursing practice. I look forward to continuing my professional development in this area of nursing practice in your program.

My enclosed résumé has more details about how my nursing practice and other academic experiences have prepared me to fulfill the needs of your staff nurse position. I would be delighted to discuss my potential contribution to your program and look forward to hearing from you.

Yours truly,

(Your signature)

Name

Enclosure: Résumé

Interview Guide

The interview provides another opportunity to market yourself. The better prepared you are before going into the interview, the easier it will be to promote yourself as the right person for the position. Thorough preparation also helps you determine whether this will be the right job for you. Your self-assessment and vision are key as you prepare for and engage in the interview process. The following three steps are a part of the interview process.

STEP 1: PREPARATION

You will need the following information:

+ Who is the employer?
+ What is the composition of the nursing team?
+ What is the job?
+ What is the interview process? Will you be interviewed by one person or a panel? If a panel interview, who will comprise the panel?
+ How long will it take?
+ Are there stages to the selection process (e.g., interview, short list, interview with committee)?
+ What is the period for decision making?
+ What is the starting salary?
+ Is the workplace unionized?

Attitude

+ Create a positive feeling about yourself and your potential.
+ Be clear about your skills and interests and how they fit with the job and the employer.
+ Identify and contact potential referees for references.

Plan

+ Develop a list of questions to ask the employer.
+ Develop a list of questions you think the employer will ask you.
+ Decide what you will wear.
+ Decide whether you will take notes with you.
+ Practise by yourself and with your mentor or a colleague.

STEP 2: THE INTERVIEW

+ Be on time.
+ Be positive.
+ Listen carefully. If you are not sure you understand the question, ask the interviewer to repeat it.
+ If you do not know the answer to a question, say so, and indicate the steps you would take to obtain the answer.
+ Remember that the interview is a two-way process; you are learning as much about the employer as the employer is learning about you.

You may be asked the following questions:

+ Describe your clinical experiences. What you have liked and not liked?
+ Why do you want this job?
+ What are your strengths and limitations?
+ Identify something you have done that you believe has worked well.
+ Identify something you would do differently.
+ What are your short-term and long-term career goals?
+ How would your colleagues describe you?

You may want to ask the following questions:

+ What are the organization and nursing department philosophies?
+ What are the goals of this unit or agency?
+ To whom will I report?
+ What are the professional development opportunities?
+ What is the employee turnover?
+ What is the orientation process?
+ How long would I work with a preceptor?
+ What is the staff mix (registered nurses, registered and licensed practical nurses, unregulated workers)?
+ What are the next steps? When will I hear from the unit or agency?

The interview usually consists of three components:

1. "Breaking the ice"
2. Having the "real" interview and gathering information
3. Closing the interview

STEP 3: FOLLOW-UP

If you are offered the position, you must evaluate the job and the offer and then make a decision. If there are some aspects of the job offer you would like to negotiate, now is the time to do so. With regard to nonunionized positions, remember that compensation includes (but is not limited to) salary and benefits.

Contact your referees and let them know how the interview went and where their references could substantiate or elaborate on your strengths.

If you are not offered the position, you may want to ask for feedback so that you can work on improving your interview skills.

An interview exercise to help you build your interview skills can be found at http://www.elsevier.ca/DonnerWheeler/

Career Planning and Development Resources: A Selected Reading List

TIP: Check your local bookstore or library for current career planning and development resources. The shelves are full. The following are good "reads" from our bookshelves.

BOOKS AND JOURNAL ARTICLES

Beatty, R. (2003). *The interview kit.* New York: John Wiley.

Beatty, R. (2003). *The résumé kit.* New York: John Wiley.

Bookey-Basset, S. (2004). Marketing yourself. In G. J. Donner & M. M. Wheeler (Eds.), *Taking control of your nursing career* (2nd ed., pp. 63–90). Toronto, ON: Elsevier.

Bolles, R. N. (2008). *What color is your parachute? A practical manual for job-hunters and career-changers.* Berkeley, CA: Ten Speed Press.

Darling, D. (2003). *The networking survival guide: Get the success you want by tapping into the people you know.* New York: McGraw Hill.

Dikel, M. & Roehm, F. (2006). *Guide to internet job searching.* New York: McGraw-Hill.

Dixson, K. (2001). Every job searcher needs an e-résumé. *Career Planning and Adult Development Journal, 17*(4), 66–78.

Donner, G.J., & Wheeler, M.M. (Eds.). (2004). *Taking control of your nursing career* (2nd ed.). Toronto, ON: Elsevier.

Donner, G.J., & Wheeler, M.M. (2007). *A guide to coaching and mentoring in nursing.* Geneva, Switzerland: International Council of Nurses.

Handy, C. (2005). *Understanding organizations.* New York: Penguin Global.

Ittelson, J. C. (2001). Building an e-identity for each student. *EDUCAUSE Quarterly, 24*(4).

Miller, T. (2003). *Building and managing a career in nursing: Strategies for advancing your career.* Indianapolis, IN: Sigma Theta Tau International.

Moses, B. (2000). *The good news about careers: How you'll be working in the next decade.* Toronto, ON: Jossey-Bass.

Rath, T. (2007). *Strengths finder 2.0.* New York: Gallup Press.

Schein, E. (2006). *Career anchors: Self-assessment.* San Francisco: John Wiley & Sons.

Simonsen, P. (2000). *Career compass: Navigating your career strategically in the new century.* Palo Alto, CA: Davies-Black.

Vallano, A. (2002). *Your career in nursing: Manage your future in the new world of health care.* New York: Simon & Schuster.

Wood, M. J., & Ross-Kerr, J. C. (2003). *Canadian nursing: Issues and perspectives.* Toronto, ON: Elsevier.

ONLINE RESOURCES

Electronic Portfolios

- Abrenica, Y. *Using electronic portfolios.* Retrieved from http://edweb.sdsu.edu/courses/edtec596r/students/Abrenica/Abrenica.html

- Lorenzo, G., & Ittelson, J. (2005). *An overview of e-portfolios.* Retrieved from the EDUCAUSE Learning Initiative Web site: http://www.educause.edu/ir/library/pdf/ELI3001.pdf

Employability Skills

- *The Conference Board of Canada employability skills.* Retrieved from http://www.calsca.com/conference_board.htm

Values Clarification

- Mensing, S. *Tips on values clarification.* Retrieved from http://www.emoclear.com/processes/values.html

- *Possible Values Clarification Exercises* (from *Instructor's resource manual for freshman orientation course*). Retrieved from Middle Tennessee State University Web site: http://mtsu.edu/~u101irm/valuesex.html

How can you be sure that you are putting you best foot forward when starting your nursing career?

In the ever-changing world of health care, what opportunities exist now and in the future?

How can you effectively plan to maximize your potential throughout your career?

Planning for your nursing career begins as soon as you enter your nursing program. *Building Your Nursing Career,* Third Edition, is a practical guide designed to help nursing students get the most out of their education and future careers, both professionally and personally. Written for nursing students at any stage of their nursing education, this guide will be an informative and helpful resource as you continue in your nursing career.

Building Your Nursing Career uses a simple model to help nursing students identify and develop their unique career goals and influence. The guide shows readers how to utilize this career planning and development model throughout their education and career. Inside, you will find useful activities and exercises to help you develop important skills you can use as you progress academically and professionally. Designed to provide practical guidance and motivating examples, it is a must-read for all nursing students who want to take charge of their careers.

Visit **www.elsevier.ca**

ISBN-13: 978-1-897422-15-1
ISBN-10: 1-897422-15-6

9 781897 422151